BRAGG

Healthy HEART

Keep Your Cardiovascular System Healthy & Fit At Any Age

PAUL C. BRAGG, N.D., Ph.D.
LIFE EXTENSION SPECIALIST

and

PATRICIA BRAGG, N.D., Ph.D.
HEALTH & FITNESS EXPERT

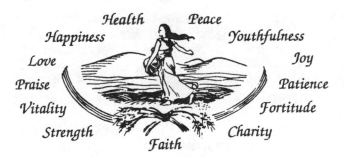

Health   Peace
Happiness   Youthfulness
Love   Joy
Praise   Patience
Vitality   Fortitude
Strength   Charity
Faith

JOIN

Bragg Health Crusades for a 100% Healthy World for All!

HEALTH SCIENCE

Box 7, Santa Barbara, California 93102 USA

World Wide Web: www.bragg.com

Notice: Our writings are to help guide you to live a healthy lifestyle and prevent health problems. If you suspect you have a medical problem, please seek alternative health professionals to help you make the healthiest, informed choices. Diabetics should fast only under a health professional's supervision! If hypoglycemic, add Spirulina or barley green powder to liquids when fasting.

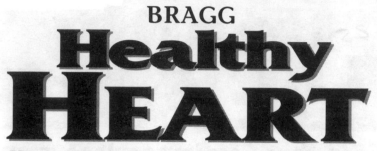

BRAGG

Healthy
HEART

Keep Your Cardiovascular System Healthy & Fit At Any Age

PAUL C. BRAGG, N.D., Ph.D.
LIFE EXTENSION SPECIALIST

and

PATRICIA BRAGG, N.D., Ph.D.
HEALTH & FITNESS EXPERT

Health Science, Box 7, Santa Barbara, California 93102
Telephone (805) 968-1020, FAX (805) 968-1001
e-mail address: books@bragg.com

Quantity Purchases: Companies, Professional Groups, Churches, Clubs, Fundraisers, etc. Please contact our Special Sales Department.

To see Bragg Books and Products on-line, visit our Website at: www.bragg.com

This book is printed on recycled, acid-free paper.

– REVISED AND EXPANDED –

Fifteenth Edition MMI
ISBN: 0-87790-096-5

Published in the United States
HEALTH SCIENCE, Box 7, Santa Barbara, California 93102 USA

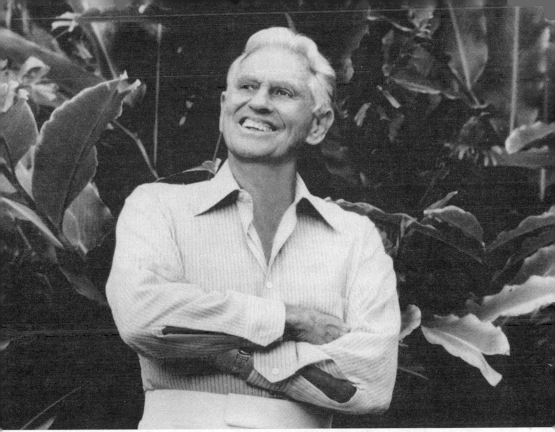

PAUL C. BRAGG, N.D., Ph.D.
World's Leading Healthy Lifestyle Authority

Paul C. Bragg's daughter Patricia and the wonderful, healthy members of the Bragg *Longer Life, Health and Happiness Club,* exercise daily on the beautiful Fort DeRussy lawn, at world famous Waikiki Beach in Honolulu, Hawaii. Membership is free and open to everyone who wishes to attend any morning – Monday through Saturday, from 9 to 10:30 am – for Bragg Super Power Breathing and Health and Fitness Exercises. On Saturday there are often health lectures on how to live a long, healthy life! The group averages 75 to 125 per day, depending on the season. From December to March it can go up to 200. Its dedicated leaders have been carrying on the class for over 28 years. Thousands have visited the club from around the world and carried the Bragg Health and Fitness Crusade to friends and relatives back home. When you visit Honolulu, Hawaii, Patricia invites you and your friends to join her and the club for wholesome, healthy fellowship. She also recommends you visit the outer Hawaiian Islands (Kauai, Hawaii, Maui, Molokai) for a fulfilling, healthy vacation.

To maintain good health, normal weight and increase the good life of radiant health, joy and happiness, the body must be exercised properly (stretching, walking, jogging, running, biking, swimming, deep breathing, good posture, etc.) and nourished wisely with natural foods. – Paul C. Bragg

i

BRAGG HEALTH CRUSADES for 21st Century
Teaching People Worldwide to Live Healthy, Happy, Stronger, Longer Lives for a Better World

We love sharing, teaching and giving, and you can share this love by being a partner with Bragg Health Crusades World-Wide Outreach. Bragg Crusades is dedicated to helping others! We feel blessed when your life improves through following our teachings from the Bragg Health Books and Crusades. It makes our years of faithful service so worthwhile! We will keep sharing, and please do write us how our teachings have inspired and helped you.

The Miracle of Fasting book has been the #1 book for 15 years in Russia! Why? Because we show them how to live a healthy, wholesome life for less money, and it's so easy to understand and follow. Most healthful lifestyle habits are free (good posture, clean thoughts, plain natural food, exercise and deep breathing that promotes energy and health in the body). We continue to reach the multitudes worldwide with our health books and teachings, lectures, crusades, radio and TV outreaches.

My joy and priorities come from God and healthy living. I love being a health crusader and spreading health worldwide, for now it's needed more than ever! My father and I also pioneered Health TV with our program "Health and Happiness" from Hollywood. Yes – it's thrilling to be a Health Crusader and you will enjoy it also. See back pages to list names (yourself, family and friends) who you feel would benefit from receiving our free Health Bulletins!

By reading Bragg Self-Health Books you gain a new confidence that you can help yourself, family and friends to The Bragg Healthy Principles of Living! Please call your local book stores and health stores and ask for the Bragg Health Books. Prayerfully, we hope to have all stores stock all the Bragg Books (we try to keep prices as low as possible) so they will be affordable and available for everyone to learn to live healthier, happier and longer!

With A Loving, Grateful Heart,

Patricia Bragg

BRAGG HEALTH CRUSADES, America's Health Pioneers
Keep Bragg Health Crusades "Crusading" with your tax deductible donations.
7340 Hollister Ave., Santa Barbara, CA 93117 USA (805) 968-1020
Spreading health continuously worldwide since 1912

ii

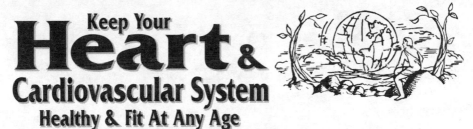

Keep Your Heart & Cardiovascular System
Healthy & Fit At Any Age

To preserve health is a moral and religious duty, for health is the basis for all social virtues. We can no longer be as useful when not well. – Dr. Samuel Johnson, Father of Dictionaries

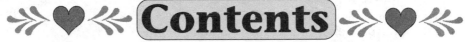

Contents

Chapter 1: Your Precious Body 1
Keep Your Precious Body & Heart Functioning at Peak Efficiency . . .1
Don't Blame Heart Attack on Hard Work, Stress, Strain or Tension .2
Primitive Humans Lived and Thrived Under Great Pressures 3
The Secret of Survival 3
Self-Preservation is the First Law of Life 4
You Can Restore Your Health & Heart 4
Ounce of Prevention Worth a Ton of Cure 5
Heart Disease is the #1 Killer 6
Your Health is Your Wealth – It's Up to You! 7
Coronary Disease is Preventable & Reversible 7
Your Powerful Miraculous Circulatory System (graphics) 8

Chapter 2: One Heart, One Life 9
Our Miracle Heart and Circulatory System 10
Important Heart Parts (graphics) .10
Our Heart is a Powerful Muscle .11
Your Hardworking Blood Network 12
For Easier-Flowing Bowel Movements 12
Eliminate the Dribbles 12
Blood Purification of Life-Giving Oxygen 13
A Healthy Heart Has Steady, Rhythmic Beats 13
The Heart Has It's Own Intelligence 14

Chapter 3: What is a Heart Attack? 15
Normal Artery Compared to Clogged Artery (graphics) 15
Be Prepared for Emergencies 16
What is Angina Pectoris? A Serious Warning! 16
The Heimlich Maneuver (graphics) 17
Heimlich Maneuver Jumpstarts Lungs & Heart (photo) 18
Heimlich Maneuver Stops Asthma Attacks 18

The Bragg Books are written to inspire and guide you to radiant health and longevity. Remember, the book you don't read won't help. Please often reread our books and live The Bragg Healthy Lifestyle for a long healthy life!

Contents

Chapter 3: What is a Heart Attack? *Continued . . .*

The Kidney's Role in Heart Attacks 19
What is a Stroke? 19
What Can You Do Today to Reduce Heart Attack Vulnerability? . .20
The Importance of Low Blood Cholesterol Levels 20
Americans Love High Cholesterol Foods .21
Some Blood Cholesterol is Normal 21
Two Types of Cholesterol – HDLs & LDLs 22
Free Radicals Are Cancer Producers 22
Free Radicals Cause Premature Ageing 23
Play it Safe – Know Your Cholesterol Levels 23
Experts State "120 to 180" Cholesterol Best 24
Fasting – Quickest Way to Lower Cholesterol 25
Cholesterol and Your Lifespan 25
How Much Fat are You Stowing Away? 25
Deadly Killer – Artery Clogging Cholesterol 26
Atherosclerosis – A Fat Hardening Disease 26
World Death Rates for Heart Disease (Chart) 27
Shocking Heart Facts About the Deadly #1 Killer 27
Cholesterol Content of Common Foods (chart) 27
Rich American Diet a Killer 28
Beware of Saturated, Hydrogenated Fats! 28

Chapter 4: Blood Pressure & Heart Attacks 29

The Silent Killer – High Blood Pressure 29
High Blood Pressure is Often Symptomless 29
What Blood Pressure Measurements Mean 30
High Blood Pressure in Adolescence 30
High Blood Pressure Linked to Mental Decline 30
Lowering Blood Pressure Reduces Heart Risk 31
AHA Says Diet Lowers High Blood Pressure 31
High Blood Pressure Drugs Pose Health Risks 32
Side Effects of Beta Blockers & Diuretics 32
Don't Procrastinate – Improve Your Health 33
Heart Surgery versus Natural Therapy 34
The Safer Road to Reduce Heart Disease .35
Non-Invasive Tests for the Heart 35
MRI– Non-Invasive Window into the Heart 36
Safer & Healthier Non-Invasive Tests For Heart Disease 36
New Millennium Health Technology Provides Better Testing 38
Dr. Paul Dudley White of Boston – Famous Heart Specialists 39
Unlimited Life Expectancy is Possible! 39
Dr. Carrel's Eternal Life Successful Study 40

Nature, time and patience are the three greatest physicians.– Irish Proverb

It's never too late to be what you might have been. – George Elliot

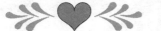 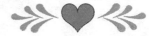

Contents

Chapter 4: Blood Pressure and Heart Attacks: *Continued . . .*

Paul Bragg & Bernarr Macfadden (photo) .41
Macfadden – Founder of Physical Culture 41
Zora Agha – Active at Age 154 42
Zora Agha's Secret of Youth 42
Zora's Longevity Diet is the Biblical Diet 43
Olive Oil Lowers Blood Pressure 43
Life's Quantity and Quality Depends Upon the Food We Eat 44
Health, Happiness & Longevity – It's up to You 44

Chapter 5: Blood – The River of Life 45

Your Bloodstream Carries Your Oxygen .45
Body's Arteries & Veins (graphic) 46
Human Life Depends on Blood 47
Teenagers Now Susceptible to Heart Disease 47
Childhood Obesity a Growing Problem 48
Early Lifestyle Triggers Obesity 49
Control Your Biological "Clock of Life" 50
"Old Age" is Not Necessary 50
You Can "Grow Younger" – It's Up to You! 51
Healthy Benefits from Eating Onions and Garlic 51
The Highway to Higher Health and Happiness 52
Risk Factors of Angioplasty on Women .52
A Healthy Body and a Happy Mind 53
Lifestyle Changes Help Remove Stress 54
AMA Says Legumes & Raw Nuts Improve Heart 54
Study Shows There's Danger in Drinking Soda Pop 54
Conrad Hilton Thanks Bragg for His Long Life! (photo) 55
It's Never too Late to Learn and Improve 55
Safer Minimally Invasive Surgery 56
Follow this Heart Health Guide Faithfully 56

Chapter 6: The Discovery of Health 57

Invest in Your "Health Bank" for Comfort, Security and Happiness 57
Start Investing in Your Health Bank 58
The "Big Three" of Health and Longevity 58
Beware of Excess Body Fat 59
Please Don't Be Overburdened With Fat 60
Your Waistline is Your Lifeline, Youthline, Dateline & Healthline . .60
Keep Trim and Fit and Your Self-Esteem 61
What is "Normal Weight?" 61
Food For Thought 62

*Open thou mine eyes, that I may behold
wondrous things out of thy law.* – Psalms 119:18

Doubt destroys – Faith builds! – Robert Collier

Contents

Chapter 7: Doctor Human Mind 63

A Sound Mind in a Sound Body .63
Correct Thinking is Important for Health 64
Your Mind Must Control Your Body! 64
Are You Poisoning Your Body? 64
A Healthy Mind for Health & Long Life 65
You are What You Eat, Drink, Breathe, Think, Say & Do 66
Drugs Control Addict's Mind 66

Chapter 8: Doctor Deep Breathing 67

When You Breathe Deeply & Fully You Live Healthier & Longer . .67
Super Breathing Improves Brain Power 68
The Lungs Are Nature's Miracle Breathers 68
You Have Lungs – Fill Them Up .69
The Importance of Clean Air to Health 70
Pollutants Threaten the Lungs of All Life 70
Live Longer Breathing Clean Air Deeply 71
Tobacco – Enemy of Your Heart and Health 72
Smoking Has Many Ways to Kill You! 72
Emphysema Smothers it's Victim .73
Vitamin C Protects Heart, Arteries & Body 74
Smoking Robs Your Body of Vitamin C 74
All Smokers – Stop Smoking Today 74
Deadly Smoking Facts (chart) 75
A Deep Desire Has Great Power .76
Be Your Body's Health Captain 76
Coffee and Non-Herbal Tea are Drugs 77
Study Shows Cola Drinks are Toxic To Body 77
Alcohol is a Depressant and Killer 78
No Self-Drugging! 78

Chapter 9: Doctor Exercise 79

Mind Over Muscle 79
Exercise Daily for a Powerful Heart 79
Enjoy Exercising – It's Healthy and Fun (Jack LaLanne photo) 80
Develope Strength for the Inside Out 81
Brisk Power Walking is the King of Exercise 81
Walk 2 to 3 Miles Daily – It Does Miracles 82
Expert Advice on How to Exercise 82
To Enjoy Your Daily Walk is Important 83

When health is absent, wisdom cannot reveal itself, art can't manifest, strength can't fight, wealth becomes useless, and intelligence can't be applied. – Herophilus

A book is a garden, an orchard, a storehouse, a party, a mentor, a teacher, a guidepost and a counsellor. – Henry Ward Beecher

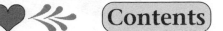 **Contents**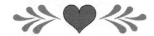

Chapter 9: Doctor Exercises: *Continued . . .*

Walking – Running – Perfect Conditioners .83
Enjoy Exercise & Jogs for Longer Life (photo) 84
Exercise is the Best Fitness Conditioner .85
Heart Disease & Irritability & Dominance 85
Exercising in the Sky – You Arrive Healthier 86
Good Shoes & Socks Promote Happy Feet 86
High Systolic Pressure in Hypertension & Heart Disease 86
Alternate Running & Walking 87
Daily Walk and Run Brings Miracles .88

Chapter 10: Exercise for Health & Good Circulation 89

Good Circulation – Key to Strong Heart 89
Five Exercises for Increased Circulation 89
Exercises – Good for Heart and Health .91
Special Shower Builds Healthy Circulation 91
Exercise to Benefit the Liver and Kidneys 92
The Dangers of Sitting too Long 92
The Art of Healthy Sitting 93
Sweating is Healthy for You! 93
Indulge in Hobbies that Are Active and Fun 94
Avoid Constricting Clothes & Shoes 94
Exercise Helps Build Better Circulation 95
Cold and Hot Water Circulation Therapy 95
Exercise Gives Benefits for Prevention of Heart Disease (list) 95
Great Framingham 50 Year Heart Study 96
Dr. T. Colin Campbell's China Project .96
Paul C. Bragg Lifting Weights (photo) .97
Iron-Pumping Oldesters (Ages 86-96 triple strength) 97
Amazing Health & Fitness Results in 8 Weeks 98
20 Year Study Shows Being Fit Saves Money 99
Wanted – For Robbing Health & Life! (list) 100

Chapter 11: Doctor Pure Water 101

Pure Water Helps Keep Body Clean Inside 101
Hard Water Causes Hard Arteries 101
Your Arteries Are Your Lifeline 102
The Difference Between Organic and Inorganic Minerals 102
Vegetable and Fruit Juices Contain Distilled Water 104
Why We Drink Only Distilled Water .105
Pure Water is Important for Health 106
The 70% Watery Human (graphic) 107

If I were to name the three most precious resources of life, I would say books, friends and nature; and the greatest of these, at least the most constant and always at hand is nature. – John Burroughs

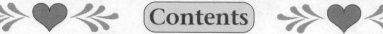

Contents

Chapter 11: Doctor Pure Water: *Continued . . .*

10 Reasons to Drink Pure, Distilled Water (list) 108
Fluorine is a Deadly Poison! 109
Keep Toxic Fluoride Out of Your Water! 109
Check Following Websites for Fluoride Updates (list) 109
Showers, Toxic Chemicals & Chlorine .110
Five Hidden Toxic Dangers in Your Shower (list) 111
Don't Gamble – Use Showers Filter That Removes Toxins 111
Toxic Exposure From Showers 112
Comparison of Water Treatment Methods (chart) 113
Foods and Allergies 114
Most Common Food Allergies (list) 114
Your Body Constantly Works for You 115
Magnesium & Calcium Vital to Heart .116
Homeostasis and the Heart 116

Chapter 12: Doctor Healthy Foods 117

Importance of a Balanced Body Chemistry 117
Protein – Building Blocks of the Body .117
Amino Acids – The Body's Building Blocks 118
Amino Acids – Life-Givers & Life-Extenders 118
Bragg Introduces Miracles of Soybeans 119
Carbohydrates, Starches & Sugars 120
Fats Can Be Healthy or Unhealthy 120
The Function of Fat in the Body 121
Low Fat Meals Cut Heart Disease Risk 121
Dr. Attwood's Tips for Low-Fat Shopping (list) 122
Dr. Charles Attwood – Great Health Crusader 122
Raw Nuts & Seeds Are Good Food 123
Organic Virgin Olive Oil Highly Recommended 124
Protective Foods – Fruits & Vegetables 124
Fresh Juices Are Best 125
The Importance of Lecithin 125
Soybean Powder for Healthy Heart & Nerves 126
What Are Live Foods? 126
Vitamin E & Raw Wheat Germ – Health Builders 127

Dr. Gerald Fletcher, a cardiologist, an American Heart Association spokesman and professor of medicine at Mayo Clinic Medical School says that "For nonvigorous activities – such as walking, pool aerobics and doubles tennis – a physician's OK is unnecessary. People can start exercising at a low to moderate intensity on their own without medical screening. Nonvigorous exercise is an activity you can do while carrying on a conversation. Remember that it's never too late to start exercising, but formerly sedentary people who begin exercising should start slowly and progress gradually, regardless of age. Even if you've been sedentary for 20 years, if you begin exercising regularly at age 50 to 60, you decrease your risk of heart disease by 25%."

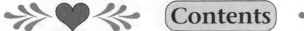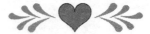

Contents

Chapter 12: Doctor Healthy Foods: *Continued* . . .

Breakfast Should Be an Occasional Meal 127
Patricia's Health Recipes 128
Vitamin E-Rich Healthy Foods (chart) 129
Calcium is Important for a Fit Heart .130
Milk is Not a Good Source of Calcium 130
Benefit From Natural Foods Rich in Calcium 131
Calcium Content of Common Foods (chart) 131
The Deadly Truth About Salt (list) 132
The Myth of the "Salt Lick" 132
Salt Affects Your Blood Pressure 133
Salt is Not Essential to Life 133
Salt is Not Necessary to Combat Heat 133
Death Valley Hike Proved Salt Dangerous 134
Bragg – the Only Non-Salt User Finished Hike 135
Break the Deadly Salt Habit! 135
What Table Salt Does to Your Stomach 136
Sea Kelp is an Excellent Salt Substitute 136
Natural Foods Have Organic Sodium 137
Your Educated Taste Buds will Guide You 137
Eliminating Meat is Safer & Healthier 138
Meat Has Toxic Uric Acid & Cholesterol 138
Vegetarian Protein % Chart (chart) .139

Chapter 13: Eat to Live - Don't Live to Eat 141

It's Harmful to Your Health to Over-Eat! 141
It's Proven – Light Eaters Live Longer 142
Food & Product Summary 143
Enjoy Super Health with Natural Foods (chart) 143
the Miracles of Apple Cider Vinegar (list) 144
Phytochemicals-Nature's Miracles Help Prevent Cancer (chart) . .145
Healthy Beverages 146
Bragg (Smoothie) Pep Drink 146
Patricia's Popcorn 146
Bragg Health Recipes 147
Avoid These Processed, Refined Harmful Foods (list) 148
Healthy Lifestyle Eating Habits (Dr. Koop photo) 149
Proper Nutrition for Rejuvenation & Fitness 150

Jesus said, "Thy faith hath made thee whole, now go and sin no more." That includes your dietetic sins! He Himself, through fasting and prayer, was able to heal the sick and cure all manner of diseases.

Relaxation techniques are very important benefits to the body's general health and cardiovascular system. Such techniques as sitting quietly, deep breathing, meditation and ignoring distracting thoughts can bring down blood pressure and are free of side effects.
– Harvard Health Letter

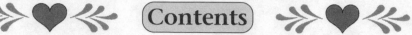

Contents

Chapter 13: Eat to Live - Don't Live to Eat: *Continued* . . .

Don't Clog Arteries with Fats & Bad Foods 150
Beware of "Killer" Foods 150
No One Need Suffer Heartburn 151
Apple Cider Vinegar Relieves Heartburn 151
Olive Oil – Mediterranean's Tasty Heart Treat 152
Folic Acid Helps Protect the Blood 153
Healthy Food Sources of Folic Acid (chart) 153
B Vitamins & Folic Acid Are Heart Protectors 154
Bragg Introduced Juicing to America 154

Chapter 14: Doctor Fasting **155**

Fasting – The Perfect Heart-Rester 155
A Story of Successful Fasting 155
Banish All of Your Fears About Fasting! 155
Cleansing the Heart Pump and Pipes .156
Flushing Poisons from your Body's "Pipes" 157
Juice Fast – Introduction to Water Fast 158
Some Powerful Juice Combinations (list) 159
Enjoy Healthy Fiber for Super Health (list) 159
Fasting Cleanses, Renews & Rejuvenates 160
Benefits From the Joys of Fasting (list) 161
Take Time for 12 Things (list) 162

Chapter 15: Doctor Rest **163**

Sound Sleep is Necessary to Build a Strong Heart 163
Sleep is Essential to Life 164
Take a Daily "Siesta" 164
How Much Sleep Do We Need? 165
Rules for Restful, Recharging Sleep 165
Your Mattress is Your Best Sleeping Friend 166
America's National Sleep Debt 167
Getting Enough Sleep Lately? 167
Before Calling it a Night 167
Try Lemon Balm for a Night So Calm .167
Tips for Healthful Sound Sleep (list) 168
For the Snorer in the House 168

---

*For most chronic conditions – like heart disease and arthritis
– exercise is a well-recognized and effective therapy.*
– Maria Fiatarone, chief of the physiology lab, Tufts University
(See how exercise improved elderly patients health on page 97 to 99.)

When one must, one can. – An Old Proverb

---

*Progress is impossible without change, and those who cannot
change their minds, cannot change anything! – George Bernard Shaw*

Contents

Chapter 16: A Frank Talk Concerning Heart Disease . . . 169

Healthy Heart Fitness Pointers (list) .170
Our Opinion of Heart Transplants .170
Heart Transplants – Risky & Costly .171
Build Yourself a Healthy Heart .172
Should the Heart Patient Always Rest? 172
Is Exertion Harmful After a Heart Attack 173
Face the Challenge – Change Your Bad Habits 174
Healthy Oils Rich in Omega 3 & Omega 6 (chart) 174
Dr. Kellogg's Famous Vegetarian Diet for Heart Patients 175
Strokes 175
Unhealthy Lifestyles=Strokes and Heart Attacks 176
Bright's Disease –Dropsy, Swollen Legs & Ankles 177
Prevention is Far Better Than Cure! 177
Pacemakers Save Lives When Needed 177
Follow This Heart Fitness Program .178
Enjoy Positive Thinking & Positive Action 178
Dr. Kellogg's Menus 179-180
Potassium Helps Strengthen the Heart 181
Potassium is the Master Mineral 181
Six Points to a Healthy Heart (list) .182
Get Close to Mother Earth & God .183
CoQ10 Combats Heart Disease, Cancer, Gum Disease, Ageing . . .183
Follow the Laws of Mother Nature & God 184
It's Up to You to be Happier and Healthier 184

Chapter 17: The Art of Longevity 185

Signs of Premature Ageing (graphic) 186
Secret of Longevity – Organized Resistance 187
Heart Disease is Your Greatest Threat 187
Old Age is Not Inevitable 188
#1 Cause of Death – Coronary Disease 189
Unhealthy Lifestyle Living is Slow Suicide 190
Your Family's Life is in Your Hands .190
Enjoy Lighter Smaller Vegetarian Dinners 191
Chinese Recipes Promote Heart Health 192
Our Favorite Chinese Recipes 193
You can Teach Old Dogs New Tricks 194
Stop Heart Trouble Before It Starts 194

Your arteries are living structures with vital functions. Their linings have about 98 different enzymatic systems, whose purpose is not only to prevent blockage damage, but to allow oxygen and nutrients to permeate freely through them into the heart muscle and other tissues. – Dr. Savely Yurkovsky, Cardiologist

Kindness should be a frame of mind in which we are alert to every chance: to do, to improve, to give, to share and to cheer. – Patricia Bragg

Contents

Chapter 17: The Art of Longevity: *Continued . . .*

Feel Youthful Regardless of Your Years 195
Paul C. Bragg & Roy D. White (photo) 196
It's Never too Late to Think Youthfully 197
We No Longer Celebrate Birthdays .197
Now Get Started – For Life is Precious 198

Chapter 18: Chelation Therapy 199

Miraculous Method of Unclogging the Arteries 199
Reversal of the "Ageing Process" 200
Beware of Deadly Aspartame Sugar Substitutes! 200
What Causes Rejuvenation & "Ageing?" 201
Chelation Therapy – Safe, Effective, Inexpensive 202
Chelation Therapy Includes a Healthy Diet 203
Safe Diagnosis with Non-Invasive Tests 203
Chelation Therapy Promotes Natural Healing 204
A Universal Need for Chelation Therapy 205
Healthy Heart Facts 206

Chapter 19: Herbs-Garlic-Supplements Nature's Healers 207

Garlic – The Herb that Lowers Cholesterol 207
Gingko – Improves Blood Flow to the Brain 208
Hawthorn – Great For Preventing Angina 208
Cayenne Promotes Healthy Circulation 209
What Are Free Radicals? 209
Life-Saving Antioxidants 210
Free Radical Catalysts Are Deadly (list) 210
B-Vitamins for a Healthy Heart 211
Vitamin C is for Capillaries & Cholesterol 211
Vitamin E – Essential for Heart Health 212
Magnesium for Your Heart, Blood & Arteries 212
Boron, Trace Minerals (graphic) 213
Words of Wisdom From Dr. James Balch 214
Words of Wisdom from Dr. Linda Page 215-218

Chapter 20: Alternative Health Therapies 219-222

A Personal Message to Our Students 223
Index 227-230

To maintain good health, normal weight and increase the good life of radiant health, joy and happiness, the body must be exercised properly (stretching, walking, jogging, running, biking, swimming, deep breathing, good posture, etc.) and nourished wisely with natural foods. – Paul C. Bragg

Living in harmony with the universe is living totally alive, full of vitality, health, joy, power, love, and abundance on every level. – Shakti Gawain

Bragg Books are silent health teachers – never tiring, ready night or day to help you help yourself to health!

YOUR BLOOD CHEMISTRY PROFILE AND YOUR HEART
By John Westerdahl, Ph.D., M.P.H., R.D.
Director of Nutritional Services and Health Promotion,
Castle Medical Center and Hospital, Kailua, Hawaii

The best way of determining your individual risk of coronary heart disease is by having a simple blood chemistry profile on a single sample of your blood. This profile should consist of five very important test values: Total Cholesterol, LDL Cholesterol, HDL Cholesterol, Triglycerides and Glucose. These tests have helped save millions of lives by alerting physicians and patients to potential health hazards in time to prevent them from occurring, by making lifestyle changes.

Many leading medical authorities state that all Americans, beginning in their teenage years, should know their blood cholesterol levels, as well as other blood values associated with heart disease! Many pediatricians say from the age of 2 on, children should have their cholesterol monitored once a year by a finger prick test. By identifying heart disease risk factors we can discover problems early and prevent them from developing into costly heart disease in years to come.

There has been much controversy over the past several years as to what the "normal" vs. "ideal" blood test values should be, especially in regards to cholesterol levels. Listed inside the front cover are what we consider the ideal values for the prevention of heart disease.

YOUNG HEALTH CRUSADER

John Westerdahl is a young Paul Bragg, for he is a dedicated True Health Crusader. He spreads the message of health throughout Hawaii via his radio talk show "Nutrition and You," and his lectures and

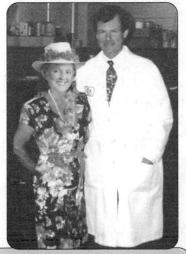

clinics on nutrition, weight control, stop-smoking, stop-drugs and his HEARTBEAT Program which promotes cardiovascular fitness. John's outreach in Hawaii has improved the health of thousands and he continues to reach millions with his world-wide health lectures, and radio programs, plus magazine articles.

John was chosen as one of the ten most outstanding young people of Hawaii. He justly deserved this high honor, for he's dedicated and loves being a health crusader! We at Health Science are proud of John. We encourage more young people into this Wellness Crusade to put America back where we belong, #1 in health and fitness instead of way down on the world list. – Patricia Bragg

Patricia Bragg with Nutritionist John Westerdahl at the famous Dr. John McDougall's Vegetarian Food Science Laboratory in S.F.

xiii

Why My Father & I Wrote This Book:

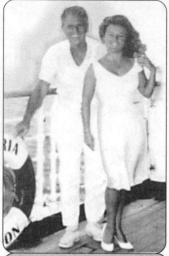

World Health Crusaders Paul C. Bragg and daughter, Patricia

Cardiovascular (heart and blood vessel) problems constitute the #1 Killer in the civilized world today. Yet these deadly problems can be prevented and controlled! Millions of our health students around the world have developed strong hearts from weak hearts. Many have averted heart surgery and helped their health and heart by living this Bragg Healthy Lifestyle and Heart Program.

My father, Paul C. Bragg, pioneered these precepts and practiced them for almost a century, with an "ageless" heart in a biologically youthful body even as a great-great-grandfather! We have both thrived on a Diet of Natural Foods all our lives. No salt, no refined white sugar or flour, no artificial additives or poisonous preservatives, no debilitating drinks, only natural "live" foods, fresh organic fruits and vegetables and their juices and distilled water combined with a Program of Healthful Exercise, Fasting, Relaxation and Revitalizing Sleep.

We want to share with you the knowledge we have gained from our years of combined experience and research so that you may no longer fear and dread the #1 Killer. You can choose to be healthy and fit and remain young in heart for your entire life! It's up to you!

🌸 Bragg Healthy Lifestyle Plan 🌸

- *Read, plan, plot, and follow through for supreme health and longevity.*
- *Underline, highlight or dog-ear pages as you read important passages.*
- *Organizing your lifestyle helps you identify what's important in your life.*
- *Be faithful to your health goals everyday for a healthy, long, happy life.*
- *Where space allows we have included "words of wisdom" from great minds to motivate and inspire you. Please share your favorite sayings with us.*
- *Write us about your successes following The Bragg Healthy Lifestyle.*

How to Keep Your Heart And Cardiovascular System Fit at Any Age

Our Active, Busy Life Sharing Health

As health experts and crusaders, we travel throughout the world teaching the simple scientific principles of The Bragg Healthy Lifestyle to millions via the media, TV, radio, and The Bragg Crusades. Every year we would personally interview, and provide Nutritional-Fitness Programs for thousands of people. Among our health students are business and political leaders, stars of the film industry, television and radio, opera, ballet and concert artists to champion athletes, etc.

As health experts, we do exhaustive research on plant, animal and human nutrition. We also supervise our organic apple orchards in conjunction with the production of Bragg Organic Apple Cider Vinegar. Our writing and working day averages 10 to 13 hours. We enjoy ample energy, exercise and tireless, ageless bodies.

Bragg Speaks About His Early Childhood

This robust health which I enjoy was acquired by the methods which are explained in this book. I was born with a weak heart, a "blue baby." Even in the modern hospitals of today, newborns with this condition must fight for their lives. I was born on a plantation deep in the heart of Virginia, in an area where cotton, tobacco and peanuts were grown and hogs were raised.

During the first 14 months of my life there was a constant struggle to survive. From infancy I suffered attacks of heart palpitation. At age 8 I was stricken with rheumatic fever and hovered between life and death for days. My life was not robust, but I had strong faith!

Having heard the word, keep it, and bring forth fruit with patience. – Luke 8:15

From Degeneration to Rejuvenation

When I was just a lad I saved a man from drowning. As it turns out this man was very rich and to reward me for saving his life he gave me a scholarship to military school. My parents were very eager for me to attend, so at the tender age of 12, I was enrolled in a large military school in the south (with a high fat, sugar diet). It was at this school that I came down with tuberculosis. I spent time in large sanatoriums, where death sentences were pronounced upon me. There seemed no hope for survival.

But where there is life (and you are still breathing) there is always hope! I was miraculously inspired by a Swiss exchange nurse at the last sanitarium to go to a famous sanitarium in the Alps of Switzerland. It was there that the renowned Dr. Rollier, who was called the "air, water, sunshine, exercise and good nutrition" doctor, used natural methods of healing to restore my sick body to buoyant, radiant health. Soon I had rebuilt my body and started climbing toward health, strength and energy!

Another important event in my life happened at this time: I made good my pledge to God at 16, that if I got my health back I would devote my life to helping others find the treasure I had found . . . Priceless, Radiant Health! Yes, that was the channel into which I wanted to direct this wonderful new energy and vitality I'd found. So many persons are forever searching blindly for "the light" – seeking health and fitness. Because I had found the miraculous formula of Natural Living, I now desired to pass on this great message to others so that they would emerge from the darkness of sickness into the crystal clear light and brilliance of Super-Health!

For decades my daughter Patricia and I have been researching longevity and natural healing methods. We have brought this message to millions worldwide. The Bragg Crusade files are filled with remarkable testimonials of what these natural methods will do to rebuild the heart and body. We now lay before you The Bragg Healthy Heart Lifestyle based on natural laws and it can do for you what it has done for us and others!

You're a Miracle – Self-Cleansing, Self-Repairing, Self-Healing – Please become aware of "YOU" and be thankful for all your blessings that take place daily!

Your Precious Body
And The Body's Miraculous Life Pump – Your Heart

Suppose a magician suddenly appeared before you and promised you a marvelous machine which could run itself, direct itself, repair itself, perform remarkable mental and physical feats . . . and would last for about 120 years and maybe more. Would you treasure such a machine? Of course you would! You would keep it in top condition in order to obtain a maximum of service. Every day you would be astonished anew by the performance of this miracle-machine!

True, this is an age of computers, biotechnology and other modern mechanical, scientific and outer space marvels. Remember that the supreme tribute we can pay to any machine is to say, *It is almost human.* Now, stop and think! Our Creator has presented you with the world's most miraculous machine – your own body! This incredible factory has its own *non-stop motor* (the heart), its own *fueling system* (the digestive system), its own *filtration system* (the kidneys), its own *thinking computer* (brain and nervous system), its own *temperature controls* (sweat glands), etc. Indeed, this miraculous creation even has *power to reproduce* itself!

Keep Your Precious Body and Heart Functioning at Peak Efficiency

Despite its importance, most of us rarely consider the care of this machine – our body – until illness strikes. By *care* we don't mean *coddling*. Instead, we mean those sensible practices and precautions which keep us in shape for the vigorous daily routine that strenuous modern living requires. Most people are fortunate to be born healthy, but far too often take this priceless gift of health for granted. Unfortunately, Mother Nature does not always let them get away with this carefree attitude. You can ruin a good car by neglect or abuse, and you can do the same with your heart and body!

Unless you know how your body functions – or malfunctions – you cannot take proper care of it. Most people's ideas about their physical processes are erroneous or far-fetched. Even in this scientific age, too many superstitions and misconceptions about the human body still persist (see page 171 – Heart Transplants).

In this book we will explain how the body works, with a straightforward account of the physical, mental and emotional factors which influence it. There will be valuable suggestions on how to keep your heart, body and its entire system running at peak efficiency.

Don't Blame Heart Attacks on Hard Work, Stress, Strain or Tension

You hear a great deal about the modern *rat race* today. You hear people saying that our *mile-a-minute* pace of living causes heart attacks. The words *hard work*, *stress* and *tension* are excuses for the rising death rates from heart attacks. (Reread Healthy Heart Habits – inside front cover.)

The basis for a heart attack is coronary blockage! The question is often asked, *Is there no warning before the blood supply to the heart begins to get dangerously low?* The answer is simple: arterial blockage grows silently and insidiously. There is usually no way of knowing exactly how much and where waste is accumulating inside one's arteries, usually until it's too late.

In some parts of the body, such as the legs, a reduced blood supply to the muscles can cause localized pain and cramping sensations. The heart sometimes gives angina pain warnings (page 16). Often there's no pain warning. This is why so many fat, flabby people, who eat any rubbish set before them will tell you they are in fine shape (no pain, problems, etc.) without taking special care of their bodies. Unfortunately, many are potentially killing themselves with their unhealthy lifestyle. When the heart attack comes, do they ever blame it on their own unhealthy habits of living? Oh, no! They blame hard work, pressures and tensions, etc!

Unhealthy cooking diminishes happiness and shortens life. – Wisdom of Ages

Primitive Humans Lived and Thrived Under Great Pressures

Let's set the record straight: humans have lived under tremendous pressure, stress, strain and tension since the dawn of history. That is what life partly is – struggle! To live is to exist under pressures of all kinds. Humans have never lived without some challenges!

In order to survive, our primitive ancestors lived under pressures that would be difficult for us to handle in today's modern world. Early humans were often the prey of wild animals seeking to kill and eat them. In times of tribal or familial wars, some humans stalked and killed one another. Wind, rain, snow and bad weather would also put them under severe duress. Humans had to survive cruel and vicious natural calamities like floods, tornadoes, earthquakes, hurricanes, plagues, famines and epidemics. In short, stress, strain and tension are nothing new to humanity. Therefore, we believe humans can face and overcome almost all of the hardest pressures life puts upon them if they are healthy, strong of body and alert of mind – this is the survival of the fittest!

The Secret of Survival

Heart trouble need not be an inevitable by-product of mounting work, stress, tension and pressures that people face daily. Though early generations had to exist under tremendous pressure, they were rugged; active physically and mentally. Their secret was simple living, natural foods (without preservatives and pesticides) and ample pure air as well as hard work, which exercises and tones the heart and muscles. As it was in the past, so it is today. Build yourself a vigorous, strong body so that you may face the great pressures of our culture today. Health, strength, endurance, stamina, vitality and energy are your protection from pressure, stress, strain and tension. Face it: this is a tough, rough, cruel and hard-boiled world in which we live. Woe to the weak for they shall perish!

Exercise reduces the risk of heart disease through direct effects on the cardiovascular system and through reduction of intra-abdominal stomach fat. The health goal of exercise and maintaining normal weight is to lower the potential for cardiovascular disease. – American Heart Association (see page 59)

Self-Preservation is the First Law of Life

This book is about having a healthy and fit heart and body. All of us must get fit for the long battle of life! There is no substitute for living a healthy life. It's up to you, whether you're rich or poor, to fight for your health and longevity with healthy eating and ample exercise!

What do we think of people who sit back and focus on making money for years while they allow their health to deteriorate? Then, when a heart attack or some other crippling ailment comes, they cry, *I have worked so hard! I have been under terrible pressure and tension! All my troubles are due to these strains.* We regard these people as uninformed and their complaints false! If they had given proper attention to their physical bodies they could have had success, money and still enjoyed health!

Hundreds of times we have heard wealthy people say, *I'd give all my wealth for my health!* If they had applied a combination of common sense and a little effort, they easily could have had both! All that is necessary is an elementary knowledge of the workings of the body and its basic needs, combined with the ability to recognize abuse and the willpower to avoid it! People spend years mastering their careers. However, devoting minutes daily learning about the health needs and limitations of their bodies seems difficult for them. **Most people tend to ignore the fact that enjoying well-earned prosperity and long, happy lives depends on their health!**

You Can Restore Your Health and Heart

One of the most remarkable miracles about the human body is its ability to repair and heal itself! For example, if you cut yourself, your body heals the cut. If you break a bone, the body heals the bone after it's set and often it becomes stronger than before. Unexpected injury may happen at any time and to *anyone*! However, if you have been taking care of your body, chances are you will recover more quickly and with less discomfort.

To preserve health is a moral and religious duty, for health is the basis for all social virtues. We can't be as useful when not well.
– Dr. Samuel Johnson, Father of Dictionaries

The less obvious injuries that we accumulate over time may also be repaired by the amazing human body. After taking a hammering for years, after being totally neglected for too long, *your body can experience astounding recovery and rejuvenation*. You must be prepared to be patient and generous with your time and effort. Just as a business that has been allowed to slip can be rebuilt. So can a neglected body! (See Conrad Hilton Story, page 55.) Don't expect a miracle overnight – *Rome wasn't built in a day*. It takes time and dedication to rebuild broken health.

Ounce of Prevention Worth Ton of Cure Towards Building an Ageless Heart

Living by The Bragg Healthy Lifestyle principles of proper diet and ample exercise promotes supreme health and longevity. Most people wait until something bad happens to their body before they do anything. We will teach you how to care for your body, so you can have an ageless and powerful heart at any age! Start today – it's priceless, exciting and fun! Challenge yourself – you will rebuild not only your heart, but your entire body!

The Bragg Healthy Lifestyle begins with nutrition. We obtain most of our energy from the food we eat, which has been directly or indirectly acted upon by the rays of the sun. Therefore, a *healthy diet* is important for the creation and maintenance of health. The next crucial step is keeping oxygen-rich healthy blood circulating throughout the body's great blood pipe system. This is accomplished with daily vigorous exercise and activity. The results will be worth all the effort you put into improving your diet and exercise. Your rewards will be a more powerful heart and a stronger body that can handle your pressures. In the end, you will welcome challenges and your healthy body and clear mind will help you overcome and solve problems wisely and successfully!

SURVIVING A HEART ATTACK WHEN ALONE (also see page 18)
Since many people are alone when they suffer a heart attack, this is very important for without help, the person whose heart stops beating properly could lose consciousness in seconds. Taking deep breaths and coughing deeply repeatedly every 2 seconds until the heart beats normally again and until help comes could save your life. The deep breaths get oxygen into the lungs and coughing movements squeeze the heart, keeps the blood circulating and helps it regain normal rhythm. www.mendedhearts.org

Heart Disease is the #1 Killer

Diseases of the heart and blood vessels take the lives of more than 1 million Americans each year – more than all other causes of death combined! In addition to being the #1 killer, it is also the #1 health destroyer. More than 60 million Americans (1 in 4) suffer from some form of cardiovascular disease. Those who survive one heart attack live in constant dread of another.

Even young children can be affected by heart disease. According to the latest studies in the Journal of the American Medical Association, atherosclerotic plaques were found in children as young as three years of age! Also, pre-atherosclerotic spots were found in half of the right coronary arteries of patients ages 15 to 19.

The chances are better than 2-to-1 that – directly or indirectly – the adult male American will die of some form of heart disease. 92,000,000 Americans living today will die of heart disease – unless they start a prevention program by living a healthy heart lifestyle.

Cardiovascular disease also affects women as well. Even though men tend to develop heart problems at an earlier age than women, cardiovascular disease rises after menopause, when levels of the reproductive hormone estrogen, plummets. After age 60, the number of women who die of heart disease is the same as men, one in four.

Be aware your lifetime savings may go straight to medical bills. Statistics reveal around 90% of American's savings goes to medical expenses especially during retirement years, if they are in poor health. Start your Bragg Healthy Lifestyle today, to ensure a bright, healthy future!

Clinical studies conducted recently by the American Heart Association show that we are almost at the point where – through proper diet and exercise – a healthy heart can be virtually guaranteed for life! Unfortunately, this truly exciting news receives relatively minor media coverage. It arouses little interest because happy and healthy people don't make big headlines.

Old age is a highly toxic condition caused by nutritional deficiencies and an unhealthy lifestyle.

Newsmen have a saying, *Great news is not interesting news*. They say it's the sensational and disastrous news that makes headlines. It's also likely that such healthy news would have raised great fury among the powerful lobbyists of the sugar, meat, dairy, alcohol, nicotine and caffeine and other unhealthy industries, who lobby heavily and spend millions on deceptive advertising.

Your Health is Your Wealth – It's Up to You!

Health, like freedom and peace, lasts as long as we exert ourselves to maintain it. It's almost exclusively in your hands whether you enjoy a healthy, vigorous life to a ripe old age or live out a half-alive, non-energetic existence with premature breakdown of health. This poor health condition predominates in *civilized* countries. Therefore, we find it ironic that so-called civilized nations are said to have a *high standard of living.* In these countries, coronary (heart) disease is the biggest killer! Apparently their *high living standards* are not producing health and longevity. See chart on page 27.

Coronary Disease is Preventable & Reversible

Dr. Dean Ornish's book *Reversing Heart Disease* states: *Heart problems are not only preventable, but also reversible by changing your lifestyle.* (Web: ornish.com) We agree – if people would only eat and exercise properly, coronary disease could be stopped in its tracks! Future heart problems would be prevented and heart disease would begin to reverse! People have the power in their own mind to take control of their lives! Most people never know real physical health. They miss out on the priceless benefits of living The Bragg Healthy Lifestyle.

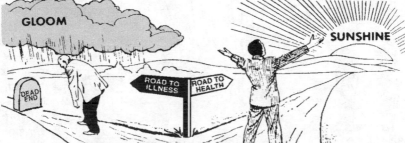

The choice of which road to take is up to the individual. He alone can decide whether he wants to reach a dead end or live a healthy lifestyle for a long, healthy, happy, active life. – Paul C. Bragg

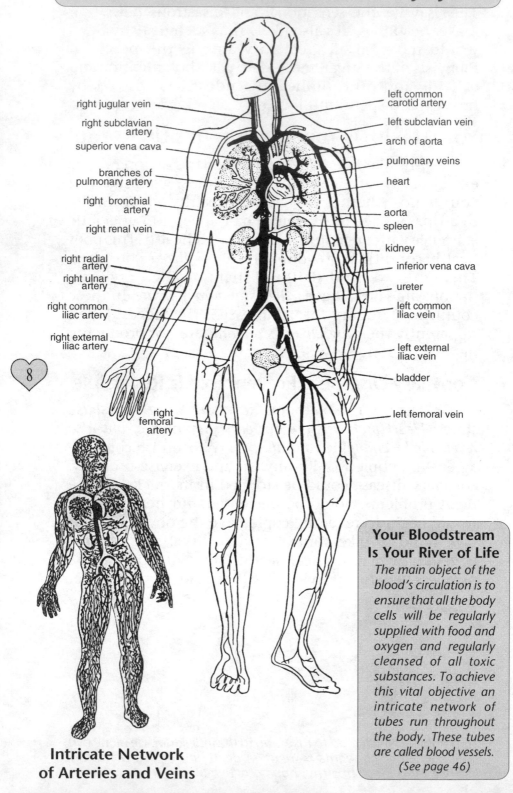

right jugular vein

right subclavian artery

superior vena cava

branches of pulmonary artery

right bronchial artery

right renal vein

right radial artery

right ulnar artery

right common iliac artery

right external iliac artery

8

right femoral artery

left common carotid artery

left subclavian vein

arch of aorta

pulmonary veins

heart

aorta

spleen

kidney

inferior vena cava

ureter

left common iliac vein

left external iliac vein

bladder

left femoral vein

Intricate Network of Arteries and Veins

Your Bloodstream Is Your River of Life

The main object of the blood's circulation is to ensure that all the body cells will be regularly supplied with food and oxygen and regularly cleansed of all toxic substances. To achieve this vital objective an intricate network of tubes run throughout the body. These tubes are called blood vessels.
(See page 46)

Chapter 2

One Heart – One Life
To Protect and Treasure

Most people are blessed with a powerful heart at birth. Of course there are always exceptions, like my father, who was born with a weak heart. He needed to fight hard just to survive. But he did survive, persevering to develop a *powerful, ageless heart* for a long life!

Your marvelous heart, the perpetual pump that Mother Nature gives us, can go on beating almost indefinitely. According to Biblical legend, Moses was 120 years old when he died; Noah was 950; Jared lived to be 962; and "all the days of Methuselah" were 969 years. Today, right here in the United States there are over 60,000 people and the count is growing who are 100 years or older. In our research on longevity we have met many people who were 100 to 115 and still living healthy lives. This shows it's possible to enjoy living a long life! What greater treasure and enjoyment is there than a long, happy, healthy, active useful life, and being kind and loving?

Truly it doesn't really matter what your calendar age happens to be. In fact, it might be better all around to forget chronological age and consider only anatomical or physiological age. *We do!* Longevity is really a vascular question. *A man is as old as his arteries.* Sir William Osler, the Canadian medical teacher and writer, pointed out long ago, *A man of twenty-eight may have the arteries of a man of sixty, and a man of forty may have vessels as much degenerated as they could be at eighty.*

Sir Osler used the word *degenerated.* Webster's defines degeneration as: *Deterioration of a tissue or an organ in which its vitality is diminished; a process by which normal tissue becomes converted into or replaced by tissue of inferior quality, whether by chemical change of the tissue (true degeneration) or the deposit of abnormal matter in the tissue (infiltration).*

Premature heart attacks unnecessarily kill almost one-half million Americans yearly. – The Stanford University Life Plan for a Healthy Heart

Our Miracle Heart and Circulatory System

At birth we are given a heart with clean arteries. It is our unhealthy foods and living habits that cause degeneration. The care we take of our heart determines the number of years we are going to stay on top of this earth. It is up to each and every one of us to take special care of our heart so we can make this life a long, healthy and happy one. Health and happiness go hand in hand.

To understand the causes of heart trouble, we must know something about the heart and the circulatory system. The primary function of this cardiovascular system (heart and blood vessels) is to distribute blood through the entire body, carrying a steady flow of nourishment and oxygen to billions of body cells. Just as important, it is responsible to remove toxic wastes from those body cells.

The blood makes its continual rounds throughout the body's 60,000 mile network of blood vessels. These vessels connect to all the body's cells, from the heart itself, to the scalp, all the way to the finger tips and toes. The average person has between *5 and 6 quarts of blood* continually circulating throughout this network. For heart facts see Franklin Institute website: *sln2.fi.edu/biosci*

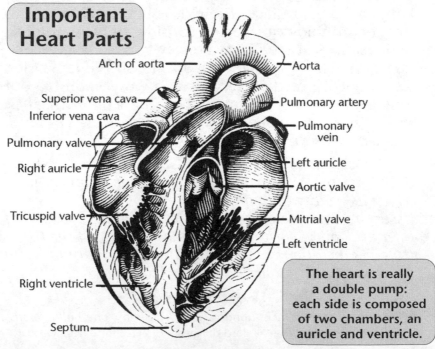

Important Heart Parts

Arch of aorta — — Aorta

Superior vena cava — — Pulmonary artery

Inferior vena cava — Pulmonary vein

Pulmonary valve — — Left auricle

Right auricle — — Aortic valve

Tricuspid valve — — Mitral valve

— Left ventricle

Right ventricle —

Septum —

The heart is really a double pump: each side is composed of two chambers, an auricle and ventricle.

Our Heart is a Powerful Muscle

The heart is not an organ of the body, it's a muscle and a very powerful, hard-working miracle! It has to be! *The heart is a muscular (double) pump* whose vital task is to pump the blood and keep it circulating in a life-long journey throughout the body. It's readily apparent that the heart has to be powerful and efficient to do all the endless work required in it's lifetime.

Consider what the heart must do: during rest or inactivity the blood makes one round trip (through the circulatory system) per minute; during activity or heavy exercise it may make as many as 9 trips a minute in order to supply the needed fuel for the increased energy and to remove the burnt-out wastes. Even during rest the heart pumps an average of 1,800 gallons of blood every 24-hours, yet it's no bigger than your closed fist.

The tissues of the body – including the heart – need oxygen to spark the chemical reaction which provides energy, just as a fire needs oxygen before it will burn and generate heat. The blood's important function is to carry oxygenated blood to nourish all the body's tissues.

The oxygen is first picked up in both lungs, then this oxygen-enriched blood (reddish in color) travels to the heart, from there it is then pumped to the tissues where the oxygen content is exchanged for waste. This blood, depleted of oxygen, turns bluish in color as it makes a return trip to the heart to be pumped back into the lungs.

Thus the heart is receiving 2 types of blood simultaneously:
- supplies of **oxygen-enriched blood** from the lungs and
- **oxygen-depleted blood** from the tissues. To keep these 2 streams separated, the heart chamber is divided in half by a muscular partition called the *septum*. The left and right chambers formed by the septum are each divided into 2 compartments. The auricle, which has a thin wall, has little pumping action and serves mainly as a reservoir. The other is the ventricle which has a thick, muscular wall and does the main pumping.

The heart pumps about 1 million barrels of blood during an average life – that's enough to fill more than 3 super tankers. – Nova Dateline

Your Hard-Working Blood Network

The object of the blood circulating is to ensure that all the body's cells will be regularly supplied with food and oxygen, and regularly cleared of toxic substances. To achieve this objective, your 60,000 mile intricate network of blood vessels run throughout your body.

The blood vessels which carry the blood *from the heart* are known as *arteries*. Those which *return the blood* to the heart are called *veins*. Both vary greatly in size, just as do streams and creeks that flow into larger rivers.

The largest blood vessel is the *aorta*, the artery which acts as the main supply pipe leading directly out of the heart and from which – through numerous branches – all parts of the body are eventually supplied with blood. The smallest tubes of both the arteries and the veins are called *capillaries* – they're so tiny that most are only visible under a microscope. Through these capillaries the last of the food and oxygen is exchanged and the return transfer is made into the veins. The veins then carry the oxygen-depleted blood and toxic wastes back to the heart for purification. On the way to the heart, most of the wastes are deposited in the kidneys for elimination from the body through the urine. Carbon dioxide, another impurity, is expelled through the lungs.

For Easier-Flowing Bowel Movements:

It's natural to squat to have bowel movements. It opens up the anal area more directly. When on toilet, putting feet up 6 to 8 inches on waste basket or footstool gives the same squatting effect. From behind use two fingers to gently pull up on edge of anus – this helps it roll out easier! Remember to drink 8 glasses of water daily! (More informaiton inside front cover.)

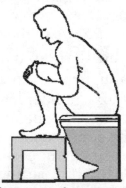

Eliminate the "Dribbles" Exercise

This will help keep the bladder and sphincter muscles tightened and toned. Urinate – stop – urinate – stop, 6 times, twice daily when voiding, especially after the age of 40. This simple exercise works wonders.

Blood Purification for Life-Giving Oxygen

When the blood – which is now full of impurities collected from the tissues of the body – returns to the heart through the veins, and then it's pumped out at once through a large artery into the lungs. There the blood sheds the carbon dioxide and absorbs the life-giving oxygen the lungs inhaled. (Don't poison this air with tobacco smoke! Read the Bragg Super Power Breathing Book.) The newly oxygenated blood then returns to the heart to be pumped out through the aorta to the body.

Blood circulation is not simple. It follows a design which resembles a figure 8. *There are actually 2 entirely separate circulations, both go away from and back to the heart.* The *greater* circulatory cycle goes to tissues, limbs, internal organs, and back to the heart. The *lesser* one goes only through the lungs and then back to the heart. Pressure in the blood vessels is naturally much greater in the arteries than in the veins, because the arteries channel the blood pumped out of the heart.

A Healthy Heart Has Steady, Rhythmic Beats

The lower part of your heart is slightly to the left side of your upper body, so it's easier to hear the heartbeat (page 114) by listening on left side of the chest. The heartbeat actually originates in the middle of the neck region and descends from the mid-line into the chest. The heart is in the center of the chest. Myths about how bad it is to sleep on your left side for fear of compressing the heart is nonsense. The best position for sleeping is on your back. (See page 166.)

A healthy heartbeat keeps a steady rhythm in its pumping, called the *pulse*. The pulse rate is usually measured at the wrist, where one of the main arteries lies near the surface. *The normal adult pulse rate is from 60-72 beats per minute.* Between each heart beat there is ⅙ of a second rest, thus when a person has lived for 50 years, their wise heart (pump) has rested 8 of those years!

Heart rate is high in newborns and declines with age, although heart rate can increase among senior citizens. Females generally have slightly higher heart rates than males. Physical activity can lower resting heart rate, which is important because a slowly beating heart is more energy efficient that one that beats rapidly.

The Heart Has It's Own Intelligence

We often hear the phrase, *I know in my heart it's true.* This indicates that we know that our heart is more than just a pump. It can beat on its own without connection to the brain. It starts to form in the fetus before there is a brain. Scientists don't know what triggers the self-initiated heartbeat. Revolutionary new heart research is emerging. The Institute of HeartMath in Boulder Creek, CA, found that the heart has its own intrinsic brain and nervous system. Fels Research in the 1970's found the *brain in the head* was dutifully obeying messages from the *brain in the heart.* The heart carries intricate messages that affect our emotions, our physical health and our quality of life! Our heart has the capacity to *think for itself.* The brain's ability to process information and make decisions is affected by how we emotionally react to a situation. (Web: *heartmath.com*)

These researchers discovered a critical link between the heart and emotions. When the heart responds to emotions such as anger, frustration or anxiety, heart rhythms become incoherent and more jagged; blood vessels constrict, blood pressure rises and the immune system is weakened. Researchers found that many heart failures were precipitated by gross emotional upsets. However, when we feel positive emotions such as love and caring, the heart rhythms become coherent and smoother; thus, enhancing healthy communication between the heart and the brain. Positive heart rhythms produce beneficial effects to cardiovascular efficiency, enhanced immunity, nervous system and hormonal balance. As we learn to become more heart intelligent and improve the emotional balance and heart/brain coherence in ourselves, we will enhance our levels of mental clarity, physical energy, productivity with more daily peace and happiness and a better quality of life.

A key factor in stress is a lack of time. In fact, 75 to 90% of all visits to physicians result from *stress-related* disorders, according to American Institute of Stress. We must utilize our time more wisely, and restore balance in our lives. Researchers found that by *locking in* to positive feelings associated with the heart, such as love, faith, joy and appreciation, we can facilitate a more perfect mental, physical, spiritual and emotional balance.

It is interesting to note that according to scientists the human brain has a storage capacity of about 1,000 years.

Chapter 3

What is a Heart Attack?

The healthy heart is a model of efficiency and perfection. When people don't watch their diet and don't exercise regularly, the walls of their arteries become cluttered with deposits of a wax-like fatty substance called cholesterol. This damages the arteries, forms scar tissue and traps more cholesterol and also mineral deposits. This condition is known as atherosclerosis. Instead of being as healthy and flexible as they need to be for the pulsing blood flow, the arterial walls become hard and brittle, since the accumulating deposits narrow the channel through which the blood must pass. All of this slows down the circulation of the blood and may even cause the formation of a clot, which blocks the blood's flow.

Normal Artery Compared to Clogged Artery
Healthy Open Artery   Cholesterol Clogged Artery

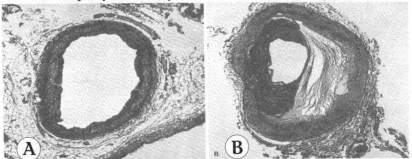

These photomicrographs show (A) a normal artery seen in cross section and (B) a diseased artery in which the channel is partially occluded by atherosclerosis.

When a clot forms in one of the arteries of the heart it creates a serious condition called coronary thrombosis, or coronary occlusion. The affected part of the heart is deprived of blood circulation. Failing to get nourishment and oxygen, it then ceases to function. This is when a heart attack occurs, and maybe even death.

Thousands of people every year pay thousands of dollars for state-of-the-art testing to learn their risk for heart disease. However, experts say that fresh vegetables and fruits and a health club membership may be better buys than any lab test. People who eat a diet low in fat and cholesterol and rich in healthy plant foods, who don't smoke, who exercise regularly, and keep their weight and blood pressure in the normal range are less likely to have a heart attack than those who don't, despite any predisposition or genetic tendency toward heart disease. – Harvard Health Letter

Be Prepared for Emergencies

Because heart attacks come suddenly, you should always be prepared for such an emergency . . . whether it happens to you or someone near you. *If you have been warned that you are a potential heart attack victim* – by your physician or by such symptoms as shortness of breath, angina chest pains, etc., it's wise for emergencies to have a portable oxygen supply, such as *Lifogen* with you. It's not heavy (3 pounds), contains 15-minute of oxygen – which is easily administered – and costs around $30, an investment that may save your life or the life of a loved one! *Safeguard, be wise and live The Bragg Healthy Lifestyle!*

Everyone should be prepared to aid a heart attack victim in an emergency; to summon the paramedics, fire department or life-guard, and to give immediate emergency treatment until professional aid arrives. The Red Cross, fire departments and schools offer courses in CPR (mouth-to-mouth resuscitation), the Heimlich Maneuver (for choking, drowning & asthma attacks) and other life-saving skills. Such knowledge may help you save lives!

(See page 123 on life-saving AEDs, automated external defibrillators.)

16

In an emergency: 1 teaspoon cayenne powder in water or juice, or cayenne tincture, (20 drops in water) may help bring a person out of a heart attack.

What is Angina Pectoris? A Serious Warning!

It's when one of the heart's arteries is temporarily deprived of blood and oxygen and goes into a spasm, causing a sharp chest pain! It's your heart's warning pain, crying for a lifestyle change to a healthy diet, fasting, exercise, etc. Usually these spasms last only a few seconds, but sometimes 3 to 5 minutes, and rarely more than 15 to 20 minutes. These are serious warnings. Please heed these warning pains listed below!

Angina chest pain is the most common symptom of heart disease, especially in women. In the Framingham Heart Study women were two times more likely to develop angina than to have a sudden heart attack as their first symptom of heart disease.

The American Heart Association advises men and women to seek fast immediate medical attention if you have any of the following symptoms:

- *An uncomfortable pressure, fullness, squeezing or pain in the center of the chest that doesn't go away in a few minutes. (Play safe: check these out.)*
- *Pain spreading to shoulders, back, neck or arms, slurred speech, ashen face.*
- *Chest discomfort – palpitations, nausea, sweating, difficulty in breathing, heartburn, feeling faint or dizzy on exertion. (See web: americanheart.org)*

The Heimlich Maneuver

First Aid for Choking & Drowning Victims & Sufferers of Asthma Attacks

(With the Victim Standing or Sitting)

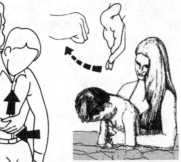

Standing in pool or water, buoyancy of water helps lighten the victim's weight.

Save a Drowning victim with the
HEIMLICH MANEUVER
You can't get air into lungs until you get water out!

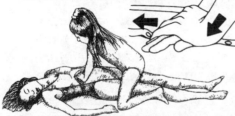

1. Stand behind the victim and wrap your arms firmly around their upper waist.

2. Place the thumb side of your fist strongly against the victim's abdomen, slightly above the navel and below the rib cage.

3. Grasp your fist with your other hand and press your fist into the abdomen with a quick upward thrust. Repeat until food/water are expelled. Do this more gently for asthma attacks.

4. If the victim is sitting, stand behind their chair and perform the Maneuver in the same manner.

5. After the victim has been revived and saved, have them see a doctor.

Note: If you start to choke when alone and help is not available, then an attempt should be made to self-administer this Maneuver.

17

First Aid when Victim has Collapsed & Can't be Lifted, Follow This Procedure:

1. Lay the victim on their back.

2. Face the victim and kneel astride the victim's hips and thighs.

3. With one hand on top of another, place heel of bottom hand on the abdomen slightly above navel and below the rib cage.

4. Press into the victim's abdomen with a quick upward thrust. Repeat as often as necessary.

5. Should victim vomit, (some do), quickly tilt head to side and wipe out vomit from mouth to prevent blocking of throat airway. (Use airway tube if necessary – keep one in first aid kit.)

6. After food, water, etc. is out, it's best a doctor check the victim.

Everyone should know the versatile Heimlich Maneuver, for it is life-saving.
– Dr. Henry Heimlich • Heimlich Institute, Cincinnati, OH • (513) 559-2391
Get radio stations to interview him. (Website: *www.heimlichinstitute.org*)

Heimlich Maneuver Jumpstarts Lungs and Heart

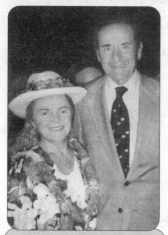

Dr. Henry J. Heimlich with Patricia Bragg in Honolulu

Pioneer Dr. Henry J. Heimlich, in 1974, developed this technique for choking victims and it has since saved thousands of lives worldwide. Recent evidence shows the Heimlich Maneuver restores breathing in more emergency situations than just choking. The Heimlich Maneuver is also handy for jump-starting the heart in heart attack victims (see www.heimlichinstitute.org); then continue with mouth-to-mouth CPR until emergency help arrives.

Heimlich Maneuver Stops Asthma Attacks

More cases are now documenting the effectiveness of the Heimlich Maneuver in stopping asthma attacks. As Dr. Heimlich explains, *"We started receiving reports from people who had suffered severe, almost deadly asthma attacks. The people who were with them didn't have any idea what to do. And off the top of their heads, they used the Heimlich Maneuver. They just tried it,"* he says, *"and immediately, instantly a miracle happened, the asthma attack stopped."*

When the diaphragm of an asthma attack victim is pushed up with the Heimlich Maneuver (whether self-applied or not), the lungs become compressed. When this happens, the trapped air is forcibly expelled and the air flow carries away the mucus plugs that started the attack. After the Maneuver, the airway is cleared and the asthma attack ends. Please share this info with asthma sufferers.

When the Maneuver is performed on asthmatics, do it gently, because you are expelling mucus and trapped air – not a stuck food object or lungs full of water. There's good evidence this maneuver can also prevent an asthma attack from occurring. Studies show applying the procedure on a regular basis helps keep the lungs free of the mucus that can plug up the airway and bring on an asthma attack. Also avoid mucus forming dairy products.

The Kidney's Role in Heart Attacks

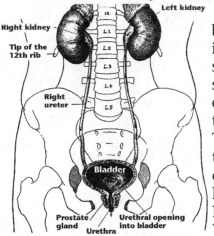

Left kidney

Right kidney

Tip of the 12th rib

Right ureter

Bladder

Prostate gland
Urethra
Urethral opening into bladder

When the circulation of blood into the kidneys is impeded, their functioning is seriously impaired. They are soon unable to efficiently eliminate the built-up toxins that accumulate in the blood. The body's vital fluid balance then gets upset and sick. This overburdens the arteries and leads to their breakdown. Millions depend on dialysis. Vitamin C and chelation helps.

What is a Stroke?

When a blood clot blocks the circulation to a part of the brain, this is what we call a *stroke*. The affected part of the brain fails to receive a sufficient supply of oxygen-enriched blood. This results in paralyzation of the part of the body that is controlled by the afflicted part of the brain. The statement, *A man is as old as his arteries*, is so true and not to be carelessly ignored!

19

Strokes are major causes of disability and death among women in their fifties and older. However, strokes can be prevented by lifestyle changes. Health education and then faithfully living it, is the best protection against having a stroke and any heart problems. *Cerebral thrombosis* is the most common type of stroke, occurring when a blood clot (thrombosis) forms and blocks blood flow in an artery supplying important blood to part of the brain. *Cerebral hemorrhage* is a type of stroke which occurs when an artery in the brain bursts, flooding the surrounding tissue with blood.

Any type of stroke is damaging, especially if the disruption of blood flow to the brain is lengthy. The brain begins to die. Then your movements can be severely restricted, as well as your ability to speak. Speech, physical therapy and hyperbaric oxygen therapy are important soon after a stroke. (See *www.strokedoctor.com*)

I've seen partially paralyzed people half carried into a hyperbaric oxygen chamber often walk out after the first treatment! – Dr. David Steenblock (800) 300-1063 CA.

What Can You Do Today to Reduce Your Vulnerability to a Heart Attack or Stroke?

There are many factors which can lead to a stroke such as: hypertension, nicotine smoking, heavy alcohol consumption, the overuse of aspirin and other drugs, and a heavy fat, salty, fried-food diet and being overweight.

Thousands of heart attacks and strokes occur every day in the U.S.! You could be next – unless you do something about it starting today! You should start immediately to prevent a future heart attack or stroke! The prevention of a heart attack is basically a life-long job of healthy lifestyle living to prevent the slow accumulation of deposits that can clog the arteries. If you are serious about avoiding a heart attack or stroke, you can begin our *Bragg Heart Fitness Program* right now.

Most cardiologists prescribe aspirin for its anti-clotting factor. They claim it may reduce heart attacks by 30% to 50% by reducing blood clotting. Caution: Aspirin may affect the clotting process too much. Also, some people may develop serious stomach problems and gastro-intestinal bleeding. What they need is immediate lifestyle changes for a healthier heart! Also, taking aspirin does not lower cholesterol or blood pressure.

So now the first thing to work for are clean arteries. The inner lining of a healthy person's arteries is smooth and flexible so that the blood can flow with ease.

Importance of Low Blood Cholesterol Levels

Every nation that lives on a modern commercial diet is eating its way into the high cholesterol danger zone of heart attacks. Evidence from studies conducted by the greatest medical authorities around the world indicates the shocking dangers of high blood cholesterol levels, see chart on inside front cover. The U.S. has the highest known average blood cholesterol level in the world, and is generally credited with the dubious honor of being the *birthplace of the coronary epidemic!* In fact, 1 out of every 2 men in the U. S. will die from a heart attack long before his normal life expectancy. This is a serious reason for Americans (especially men) to take action right away!

Americans Love High Cholesterol Foods

American men love all these cholesterol disasters: steaks, big slices of roast beef, thick slices of ham, ribs, pork chops, fried chicken, roasts, bacon and luncheon meats, as well as cheese, ice cream, whipped cream, cream, sour cream, milk, butter, eggs, commercial pies and pastries, candy, french fries, meat gravies, potato chips and commercial salad dressings made with saturated oils.

All these favorite American foods have a lot of *hard or saturated fats,* primarily of animal origin. These saturated fats are *high in cholesterol.* Consequently, the average blood cholesterol index in the United States today is between 230 and 260 – far above the *safety level.* High blood cholesterol levels have definitely been established as the *forerunners* of most heart attacks.

It is perfectly normal to have a certain amount of fat and cholesterol in your bloodstream. Called *lipoproteins,* they are necessary for the upkeep of the body. However, trouble begins when you have an excess of fat clogging your body's pipes. This is why it's essential to master and live The Bragg Healthy Lifestyle; it helps keep your blood cholesterol levels healthy and normal.

Some Blood Cholesterol is Normal

Every cell in the body needs some cholesterol to function properly. Produced in the liver, cholesterol is delivered through the bloodstream to all the various cells of the body. However, the cells take only what cholesterol they need; any excess remains in the bloodstream. The unused cholesterol eventually collects in the circulatory system as plaque deposits that clog artery walls.

Good news – the liver rarely produces more cholesterol than the body needs. The bad news is that it can enter the body by more ways than the liver's activity. What you eat also greatly influences your cholesterol levels!

Let Mother Nature wisely help you keep the doctor away. Researchers in the Netherlands have found that people who lovingly tend to houseplants or a small flower or vegetable garden have significantly fewer heart attacks than people who don't. Gardening was also found to lower blood pressure. So plant an organic veggie garden today for more blessings of health and happiness.
– Patricia Bragg, an ardent organic gardener and fan of organic foods!

This fatty substance, cholesterol, is found in the liver, brain, nerves, bile and blood of all humans and mammals. Eating meat and dairy products can adversely raise your cholesterol levels. Because when this is beyond the amount your body needs, the excess remains in the bloodstream and collects along arterial passages. Warning: this arterial cholesterol buildup may cause serious cardiovascular blockage and even death!

Two Types of Cholesterol – HDLs & LDLs

RESEARCHERS DISCUSS THE 2 MAIN CHOLESTEROL TYPES:

FIRST are the *high-density lipoproteins (HDLs)*, known as *good cholesterol*. High HDL levels are linked to a lower risk of heart disease and heart attack. Researchers believe that HDLs travel through the bloodstream collecting *bad cholesterol*. But the exact benefits of HDLs are difficult to estimate, because after the HDLs have traveled through the bloodstream they may return to the liver and be turned into bad cholesterol!

SECOND are the *low-density lipoproteins (LDLs)*, often referred to as the *bad cholesterol*. When LDLs occur in excess in the body, they dangerously coat and clog arterial walls. LDL cholesterol is also very dangerous in another way: when exposed to heat and oxygen, these cholesterol molecules slowly change. When it occurs in fats, we call this process *going rancid*. When fats go rancid, their LDLs become infested with *harmful free radicals*.

Free Radicals Are Cancer Producers

Free radicals (cancer producers) are very dangerous elements that alter and change food molecules. With LDLs (found in all animal proteins and their by-products), free radicals change the original cholesterol structure into more than 400 different harmful, toxic substances! Once in the body, free radicals roam widely, attacking and damaging cells. Free radicals are introduced into the body through your environment as well as by your diet. See the *Free Radical Catalysts* list on page 210.

Cardiovascular disease is not the inevitable result of ageing. Preventative measures can be taken to avoid heart disease. – James F. Balch, M.D.

Free Radicals Cause Premature Ageing

Most risk factors for coronary heart disease, such as high blood pressure or smoking, create free radicals that prevent the inner walls of blood vessels from producing nitric oxide. This is necessary for proper blood vessel expansion and contraction. A free radical is an unstable molecule, that reacts with other molecules in destructive ways! An excess of free radicals causes premature ageing and serious medical conditions, depending on which tissues are being attacked. The free radicals may attack DNA (your genetic inheritance) causing cancer or even birth defects; in the pancreas they can cause diabetes; if in the eye they can cause cataracts, and in the blood and blood vessels they can cause cardiovascular disease.

Don't be a passive victim of destructive free radicals! Take heart, avoid the unhealthy foods we have listed on page 148. Living The Bragg Healthy Lifestyle helps arrest free radicals and ageing, and earns you a healthier heart and body for enjoying a longer, healthier life! Faithfully guard and protect your precious body and health!

23

Play it Safe – Know Your Cholesterol Levels

There are many simple home cholesterol tests now widely available. These FDA approved tests are over 97% accurate and require only a fingerprick. The test kit cost is between $10 to $20, and available in most drug stores. See options on web: shoptheplaza.com and testathome.com

When you have a complete cholesterol panel ask your doctor for a copy of your HDL, LDL and triglyceride levels. These readings determine your main risk factors for heart disease. HDL *good* cholesterol helps protect you from a heart attack. You can help raise your *good* HDL by eating healthy foods, exercising and losing any excess weight and quitting smoking. An HDL less than 35 mg-dl puts you at a health risk. The LDL or *bad* cholesterol should not exceed 130 mg-dl. To lower undesirable LDL levels, seek a low-fat, low-cholesterol, low-saturated fat diet. Triglyceride levels over 200 mg-dl, are dangerous and associated with obesity, sweets, fats and alcohol intake.

(For Recommended Blood Chemistry Values see inside front cover.)

- Consume less than 300 mg of cholesterol per day.
- Consume 30% or less calories from fat.
- Consume 10% or less calories from saturated fat.

If you want to keep your daily cholesterol count, you may purchase a fat gram counter which counts cholesterol, total fat and saturated fat in foods. We personally don't count calories, fat grams, etc. We live our Bragg Healthy Lifestyle and it keeps us healthy. But while you are learning this healthy lifestyle you can count grams if you have the time. Be aware that cholesterol can accumulate in the skin and tendons, as well as the arteries, to form small flat yellow plaques and lumps called xanthoma. The plaques found on the eyelids produce a condition called xanthelasma.

Follow these golden rules for maintaining safe cholesterol levels: eat only healthy, natural foods; get plenty of exercise; breathe deeply and fully; drink 8 glasses of pure distilled water daily; and get 8 good hours of sleep nightly. Those of you who are at any high risk of cardiovascular problems – caution, please take extra care to be aware of your current blood cholesterol levels. (See chart on inside front cover for safe cholesterol ranges.)

Experts State "120 to 180" Cholesterol Best

Top medical scientists and researchers agree that a person's blood cholesterol level should not be over 180. Here are some professional opinions:

- *"150 to 180,"* according to Dr. W. D. Wright of the University of Nebraska College of Medicine.
- *"170,"* was the opinion of Dr. A. G. Shaper of the Makerer College Medical School in Uganda.
- *"180 as a maximum,"* stated Dr. Bernard Amsterdam in the New York State Journal of Medicine.
- *"150,"* according to famous Dr. Louis H. Nahum of the Yale School of Medicine.
- *"120 to 180,"* is optimal normal range stated Dr. William Dock, Professor of Medicine, State University of New York.

Fasting – Quickest Way to Lower Cholesterol

In our opinion, fasting is the quickest, easiest and fastest method of lowering the cholesterol level. We check our blood cholesterol twice a year. If it tops 180, we fast from 3 to 7 days and it soon drops below 150. Fasting (pages 155-161) is an easy way to give the heart and cardiovascular pipes a good cleansing. That's why faithfully each week we fast for a 24-hour period on 5 to 7 glasses of distilled (purified) water and also three Bragg vinegar drinks (page 146). For more details on the Science of Fasting, read our book *The Miracle of Fasting*. See book list on back pages for ordering.

Cholesterol and Your Lifespan

One thing that will unquestionably shorten the lifespan is a body that is overburdened with blood fat, an excess of cholesterol. To reiterate: some cholesterol is important to our body processes. The body even manufactures it as extra fuel in emergencies. *Chole* means bile and *sterol* means fatty. Much of the fat we eat is broken down by the liver into cholesterol and excreted into the bile, later to be re-absorbed into the bloodstream for distribution to our tissues.

How Much Fat Are You Stowing Away?

Too many people today eat a diet overloaded with the high cholesterol content of saturated (hard) animal fats. When these people increase the burden on their bodies by not exercising enough to burn up even the normal – much less the excess – amount of cholesterol as fuel, their bloodstreams become *choked*. Waxy cholesterol particles lodge in the arterial walls and clog them. These chunks of waxy cholesterol can eventually block an artery and cause heart failure, stroke or death!

It has been clinically established that the amount of cholesterol deposited on the walls of the arteries has a direct relationship to the amount of cholesterol in the bloodstream. Thus you can see how clogged the arteries must be when the blood cholesterol level rises to 270, 320, 380 and even higher! Yet these excessive levels are not uncommon today, especially in American men.

Deadly Killer – Artery Clogging Cholesterol

Remember that the amount of cholesterol in your blood tells you of the risk you are running of developing a coronary ailment or having a heart attack. It is *the barometer of your life-span.* It is very wise, therefore, for every adult to see to it that they do not raise their blood cholesterol above a safe, normal level.

Most people know little or care nothing about their cholesterol levels. They merrily go on using large quantities of butter on their bread, toast, potatoes and vegetables. They drink great quantities of milk and gobble gallons of ice cream and meat, fish, poultry, eggs, chips, french fries, doughnuts, bacon, ham and sausage – all fill their bloodstreams with excess fat! Little do they realize their high levels of cholesterol are leading them to disaster, and that they may be literally eating themselves to death! Millions of people consume as many as 4 or 5 cups of saturated fats daily. Then they wonder why they end up with a heart attack, stroke or some other form of heart trouble – it's clogged arteries!

Atherosclerosis – A Fat Hardening Disease

As mentioned previously, the clogging of the arterial system by excess cholesterol – the deposits of heavy, waxy fat on the artery walls – is called *atherosclerosis.*

The components of the word, *atherosclerosis*, are of Greek origin. *Athere* means porridge or mush and refers to the soft fatty material in the core of the plaque; *skelros* means hard and refers to the hard scar-like tissue formation involved in the development of a plaque, and *osis* is a greek suffix meaning a diseased condition. Therefore, it's a fat hardening disease.

The term arteriosclerosis is a group of diseases that cause thickening and blocking and loss of elasticity of the artery wall. Both atherosclerosis and arteriosclerosis are often used interchangeably. Atherosclerosis most frequently affects the aorta – the largest blood vessel in the body, the coronary arteries and cerebral arteries which supply the brain, the legs and abdomen. Atherosclerosis is initiated by high blood pressure, smoking and increased concentration of fats in the bloodstream.

World Death Rates Due to Heart Diseases From Fat in Diet

Country	Women Death Rate Per 100,000	% Fat in Relation to Total Calories
Finland	314	39.2
United States	323	31.1
Canada	229	38.0
Australia	250	37.9
New Zealand	389	39.8
United Kingdom	354	38.4
Germany	299	35.6
Denmark	306	38.3
Sweden	235	39.4
Austria	311	31.3
Switzerland	167	33.6
Belgium	225	35.0
Norway	266	38.0
Italy	213	22.3 *
France	131	29.5 *
Portugal	312	24.5 *
Japan	161	7.9 *

*This chart illustrates the striking difference between Finland and Japan, the death rate varying by more than 250%. * Lowest 4 countries use less saturated fats. – American Heart Association*

Shocking Heart Facts About the #1 Killer

27

- Cardiovascular diseases claimed over a million lives in the United States last year, accounting for almost half of all deaths!

- Every 33 seconds another American dies from cardiovascular disease!

- Heart disease doesn't just kill the old; 1 out of every 6 is under 65!

- Heart disease affects both men and women; lately men accounted for 49% of heart related fatalities, while women accounted for 51%.

Don't let cardiovascular disease affect you! Protect your heart!

CHOLESTEROL COUNT OF COMMON FOODS

FOOD FROM ANIMAL

Cholesterol Count	(mg)
Brain, 3oz	1,749
Liver, chicken, 1 cup	883
Liver, beef, 3oz	331
Kidney, beef, 3oz	329
Butter, 1 pat	250
Egg, whole	213
Cream cheese, 8oz	120
Ice cream, 1½ cup	88
Lamb, 3oz	78
Beef, sirloin steak, 3oz	77
Pork, 3oz	77
Chicken breast, 3oz	73
Chicken leg, 2oz	48

FOOD FROM PLANT

Cholesterol Count	(mg)
All beans	0
All fruits	0
All grains	0
All legumes	0
All nuts	0
All seeds	0
All vegetables	0
All vegetable oils	0

Sources:
1. J. Pennington, Food Values of Portions Commonly Used
2. Family and Consumer Service, University of Georgia
www.fcs.uga.edu/pubs/current/C761-06.html

Rich American Diet is a Killer

Atherosclerosis is not brought on by age, but by diet! Autopsies of the American soldiers killed in battle in the Korean War revealed the shocking fact that 77% of these soldiers (average ages 18-22) already had atherosclerosis! In contrast, the Koreans and other Asians who died on the same battlefield, under the same conditions, had only an 11% incidence of this disease. It's well known, the traditional Asian diet is low in saturated fats.

The U. S. is a nation of fat-eaters. Saturated fats make up 40% of the caloric intake of the average American diet. Most of these are the commercial, hydrogenated fats – the most clogging, deadly of all fats and are not natural in any sense of the word. It's such a solid fat that it cannot be broken down by the body's 98.6°F heat.

The best natural, unsaturated fats break down at body temperature and don't cause clogging problems. These are perishable foods and don't have a long shelf life. In time, these unsaturated fats take on oxygen and become rancid, which gives off a strong odor and bitter taste.

Beware of Saturated, Hydrogenated Fats!

Hydrogenated, saturated fat remains *stable* because it's impervious to oxygen. In reality, it is embalmed fat! The American consumer has been brainwashed by the greedy, large manufacturers into believing that they are permanently fresh and healthy! A container of this processed fat will keep in the house for years, because it's impossible for it to turn rancid. Clever advertising says these saturated, hydrogenated, snow white, processed (erroneously called vegetable) shortenings will not smoke. They also make other clever sales claims which have no relation whatsoever to good nutrition. The same applies to unhealthy margarine made to imitate butter.

So – instead of the natural, unsaturated fats that will aid health – Americans consume deadly hydrogenated, saturated fats, high in cholesterol that coats and clogs the bloodstream, especially the vital arteries. All this clogging eventually causes fatal or crippling clots (thrombosis) into the bloodstream, causing strokes.

Chapter 4

Blood Pressure & Heart Attacks

The Silent Killer – High Blood Pressure

What happens when you blow too much air into a balloon? If it doesn't pop, the overextended balloon becomes thin and delicate. Properly inflated, the balloon can be safely bounced, bent and moved around. A balloon with too much air becomes a pop waiting to happen. Don't let this happen to your vessels and heart.

We need blood pressure for our blood to circulate. Too much pressure makes the heart and blood vessels thin and delicate. Increased pressure on the arterial walls makes them more susceptible to fatty deposits.

High Blood Pressure is Often Symptomless

The dangers of untreated hypertension can be deadly! If left untreated, the arteries can become hardened, scarred, and less elastic, unable to carry adequate blood to the organs. The heart, brain and kidneys are most vulnerable. High blood pressure is the highest risk factor for stroke and heart disease. High blood pressure causes the heart to enlarge and become less efficient, known as left ventricular hypertrophy. This dangerous condition can lead to heart attacks. Many connect stress with high blood pressure. Some studies have suggested that chronic stress can lead to permanent increases in blood pressure and heart rate. Example: air traffic controllers who have high-pressure jobs, have a two to four times higher rate of hypertension and heart problems.

For a healthy, fit heart, it's wise to keep your blood pressure within the normal 120/70 range. You can manage this with simple dietary and lifestyle changes. Exercise, deep breathing, ample sleep and a healthy diet helps keep your blood pressure under healthy control.

Don't eat salt or add salt to food, and avoid prepared foods with high salt, sugar and fat contents. Especially avoid simple sugars like refined sugar and *keep your fat intake to a minimum!* Never use highly saturated fats. Avoid the fast, nutritionally empty foods so common in our *on the go* culture. *Eat nutritious foods!*

29

What Blood Pressure Measurements Mean

There are two types of blood pressure readings. *Systolic* pressure (first figure in reading) refers to pressure exerted by the blood while the heart is pumping; this reading indicates blood pressure at its highest. D*iastolic* pressure (second figure) reads the blood pressure when the heart is at rest in between beats, when the blood pressure is at its lowest. Both readings are important; neither should be high. A normal pressure reads 120 over 70 to 80 (120/70-80), with the systolic pressure measuring 120 mmHg and the diastolic pressure measuring 70 to 80 mmHg.

High Blood Pressure in Adolescence

New Millennium Studies presented at the Scientific Session of The American College of Cardiology in Anaheim, California, found that children who are overweight at ages as young as six or seven, are more likely to have high blood pressure by adolescence! Researchers studied 200 children for ten years, examining blood pressure, obesity and metabolic abnormalities. The results showed the body mass index (overweight) correlated strongly to higher blood pressure in the children, even after they reached young adulthood. The finding strongly suggests primary overweight prevention may need to begin even before the first day of school, promoting good nutrition as well as exercise and fitness.

High Blood Pressure Linked to Mental Decline

High blood pressure can lead to declines in some mental abilities, according to researchers at the University of Maine (*http://www.docguide.com*). *Elevated blood pressure is a strong predictor of changes in brain structure and related cognitive functioning.* The researchers examined blood pressure and mental function in 140 men and women age 40 to 70 years old. They found that higher levels of blood pressure was associated with greater declines in intelligence tests, visual-spatial abilities and speed of performance.

Harvard School Public Health Study found 84% of those who sought a second opinion after scheduling heart bypass surgery, were told they didn't need it!

Many patients who undergo heart bypass surgery suffer a significant and long-lasting loss of brain power. For the full story on this alarming news, see www.nim.nih.gov/medlineplus/news/fullstory146.html

Lowering Blood Pressure Reduces Heart Risk

The International Society of Hypertension unveiled results of the largest hypertension study ever completed, called the Hypertension Optimal Treatment (HOT) study, they found lowering diastolic blood pressure level of 90 mmHg, can help reduce major cardiovascular risk! The study also found that patients with diabetes, who lowered their diastolic blood pressure level to 80 mmHg, lowered their risk of cardiovascular problems. This study amassed 18,790 patients in 26 countries over a five-year period. According to Dr. Claude Lenfat, director of the National Heart, Lung and Blood Institute, *If physicians lower blood pressure beyond traditional levels of 90 mmHg, there's reason to believe that cardiovascular morbidity and mortality can be diminished.* The study found that patients with coronary artery disease, had a 43% reduction in strokes with those whose blood pressure level was a healthier 80 mmHg and lower. High blood pressure (hypertension) is the most common heart disorder and a leading cause of death in America. Over 300,000 deaths per year in persons age 65 to 84, are due to cardiovascular disease and more than $259 billion dollars are spent for their medical care!

AHA Says Diet Lowers High Blood Pressure

Individuals with high blood pressure should not only put away the salt shaker, but eat more fruits, vegetables and fat-free or low-fat dairy products, announced the American Heart Association's nutrition committee. They also recommend potassium, calcium and magnesium rich diets. Dr. Theodore Kotchen, AHA nutrition committee member stated, *This indicates that dietary components other than salt are also important in the control of high blood pressure. Diets which are high in potassium such as bananas, dates, potatoes and raisins tend to lower blood pressure.*

We tend to think of advances in medicine as being a new drug, a new surgical technique, a new laser, something high-tech and expensive. We often have a hard time believing that the simple choices that we make each day in our diet and lifestyle can make such a powerful difference in the quality and quantity of our lives, but they most often do. My program consists of four main components: exercise, nutrition, stress management, love and intimacy – these promote not only living longer, but living better. – Dean Ornish, M.D.

One in four American adults have high blood pressure, which increases their risk of stroke, heart attack and kidney failure. *Avoiding a high-salt diet, not being overweight individuals and restricting alcohol intake are very important,* notes Dr. Kotchen.

High Blood Pressure Drugs Pose Health Risks

When it comes to dealing with high blood pressure, most Western doctors turn first to drug treatments. They rely mainly on pharmaceuticals – *diuretics* and *beta-blockers*. Drug *diuretics* (with side effects) lower blood pressure by reducing the volume of blood. With less blood, pressure in the arteries decreases. The other commonly prescribed type of drug, the *beta blocker,* (also with side effects), works on the autonomic nervous system. Beta blockers slow the heart rate, which reduces pressure by reducing the amount of blood the heart pumps.

Side Effects of Beta Blockers and Diuretics

These both claim to be helpful remedies for high blood pressure, don't be too sure. **Diuretics** relieve one problem only to give rise to several others: They deplete blood of certain essential minerals, increase blood's cholesterol level, and increase blood's thickness, stickiness and acidity. These factors increase heart attack or stroke risk. Studies show that death rates increase with heavy diuretic use.

What about **beta blockers**? Though their cardiovascular side-effects are less pronounced than with diuretics, beta blockers are known for causing impotence, depression and fatigue. Because their job is to make the heart lazy and slow, beta blockers ensure that the hands, feet and brain get less blood and less oxygen!

You can avoid these dangerous drugs and maintain a healthy blood pressure at the same time. Take the advice of a growing legion of progressive medical practitioners who treat high blood pressure without dangerous drugs. Doctors like Alexander Leaf of the Harvard Medical School, and William Roberts, editor of *The American Journal of Cardiology,* recommend making lifestyle changes rather than drug prescriptions for high blood pressure patients.

Our habits, good or bad, are something we can control. – Dr. E. J. Stieglitz

Don't Procrastinate – Improve Your Health

What kind of lifestyle changes are best? Those that instill the health habits we teach with The Bragg Healthy Lifestyle! A low-fat, vegetarian diet is crucial for the free and unimpeded flow of blood through your body. Reducing fat in your diet also stimulates weight loss, which, in turn, contributes to reduced blood pressure. Finally, make exercise a fixed part of your daily routine and learn to breathe deeply and relax, freeing yourself of stress while you fill yourself with ample fresh oxygen. Begin today to make this Bragg Healthy Lifestyle a lifelong happy habit! It is bringing miracles to millions.

Please listen to Dr. Claude Lenfant, Director, National Heart, Lung & Blood Institute. He says *Lifestyle changes alone can actually reverse the conditions of heart disease.* When it comes to making the kind of changes needed for healthy and happy living, the truly important thing is making those changes happen. However, actually doing it, living it, making it happen – this is what counts! So don't play procrastinating games with yourself! The moment you think, *Do I have time to do this right now?* is the moment to stop asking and start doing. The moment you think, *I want a big steak for dinner*, is the time to open up a vegetarian cookbook with pictures and discover healthy, tasty new recipes. We promise you will find recipes more delicious, healthy and satisfying than steak. If you do eat meat, limit it to 1 to 3 times a week and be sure it's hormone-free and organically fed without harmful chemicals.

Millions of successful Bragg students will tell you the same thing: the beginning is the most difficult. The in-between moment after you decide you want to become healthier and before you begin to act on that decision, is the hardest. Example: the moment before you put one leg in front of the other on the first step of your brisk walk is the hardest moment of the exercise.

Love is the sun shining in us to sparkle our lives! – Patricia Bragg

Dr. Dean Ornish has been able to reverse heart disease in more than 70% of his patients who follow, among other things, a low-fat vegetarian diet.

Once you dedicate your life to health and fitness you're living The Bragg Healthy Lifestyle – your Fountain of Continual Youthfulness! Soon you will look forward with joy to your daily exercises. Also, you will wonder how you could ever have eaten the unhealthy and unappetizing foods that once half-way sustained you. Plan, plot and follow through with The Bragg Healthy Lifestyle living. Getting started is what counts. Start Now!

Heart Surgery Versus Natural Therapy

Unfortunately, our Western medical professionals too often turn first to invasive procedures rather than safer and less expensive non-invasive, healthier alternatives. This is true in both diagnosis and treatment.

An *angiogram* is an invasive and dangerous diagnostic test (causes approximately 20,000 deaths yearly) that is supposed to measure blood flow and blockages in the heart. A catheter is inserted into a patient's leg artery (through the groin), and threaded up through the artery all the way to the patient's heart. A National Heart, Lung & Blood Institute study found this painful invasive procedure is a shocking 82% inaccurate! Nevertheless, doctors continue to prescribe expensive angiograms. In the years since the study, angiograms performed in the U.S. have risen from 380,000 to well over one million yearly!

Expensive treatment for heart disease is increasingly dominated by invasive procedures. In the 17 years between 1979 and 1997, coronary bypass surgeries increased a shocking 432% – from 115,000 operations to 607,000 performed yearly! If only this trend reflected a growing, positive effectiveness of these invasive procedures – but this is not the case! These and current studies prove it!

A recent Harvard University medical study reports that invasive heart surgeries have little effect on the long-term survival of most heart patients. Only in the most severe cases did dangerous, invasive operations show significant statistical merit. The study suggested that these types of surgeries could be reduced by 25% or more without endangering the health of heart patients. Rather than using this important study's advice, doctors are increasing expensive heart surgeries at an alarming rate!

The Safer Road to Reduce Heart Disease

Dr. Julian Whitaker, one of America's famous heart specialists, became so outraged years ago over unsafe trends that, as he says, *I gave up being a surgeon to become a healer.* He founded the renowned Whitaker Wellness Institute in Newport Beach, California, and has the nation's leading health newsletter, *Health and Healing.* A healthy lifestyle like The Bragg's Lifestyle is his alternative to angiograms and surgery. *www.drwhitaker.com*

Dr. Dean Ornish, the Clinical Professor of Medicine, School of Medicine, UC San Francisco, is another world famous doctor-turned-healer. When Ornish's heart patients embraced a healthy, energetic exercise regime and ate only nutritious, low-fat foods, their heart conditions began improving within one month! After a year, most patients had virtually no chest pains or heart problems! For 82% of his patients a healthy lifestyle reversed their arterial clogging! Web: my.webmd.com

Non-Invasive Tests for the Heart

The safer, less expensive, non-invasive alternatives can bring about greater health. The invasive heart tests and operations are extremely dangerous, expensive and often unnecessary! There's a growing number of doctors that specialize in protecting heart patients from the use of angiograms, bypass surgery and angioplasty. As an alternative to invasive testing procedures, they place sonar devices, electronic sensors, microphones, etc. on the outside of the chest. These sensitive tests can usually judge heart disease better than procedures which use dangerous, invasive catheters, tubes and needles.

When needed, consult with some of the many physicians and health organizations working to make the healthcare of your heart a wise, safer job. Here's some sources:

❤ **The Whitaker Wellness Institute**, Newport Beach, CA (949) 851-1550 • *www.whitakerwellness.com*

❤ **Dr. Dean Ornish**, PMRI Institute, CA • For Heart Retreats (800) 775-7674 X221 • *www.pmri.org* or *my.webmd.com*

❤ **ACAM** (American College for Advancement in Medicine) (800) 532-3688, for CA and Foreign (949) 583-7666. For list of holistic doctors see web: *www.acam.org*

MRI – Non-Invasive Window into the Heart

Doctors use *magnetic resonance imaging* (MRI) as a non-invasive, diagnostic tool to look at the soft tissue inside of a patient without having to invade the body. MRIs use a powerful, but harmless magnetic field that reveals in great detail the shape and condition of your internal organs. Doctors can use this test to diagnose various conditions of the heart and the entire body.

What can this non-invasive MRI procedure tell a doctor about a patient's heart and circulatory system? *Miracle* MRIs can identify heart scarring and any other indications of a previous or future heart attack. It can reveal arterial clogging and the presence of other foreign masses in, and around, the heart and body. It detects any signs of heart disease, identifies vascular disorders and checks blood vessel health. Warning: MRIs cannot be used on people with pacemakers or arterial clips.

Safer and Healthier Non-Invasive Tests For Heart Disease:

DOPPLER COLOR FLOW IMAGING TEST This is a safe, non-invasive imaging ultrasound. It shows a clear profile that checks the entire blood vessel system simultaneously. When needed, doctors check for possible blood slow-down and blockages that can cause future heart attacks and strokes, and even death. *www.dvonch.com/doppler.html*

ELECTROCARDIOGRAM & CARDIOKYMOGRAPHY It's an EKG and CKG graph that records electrical activity in the heart. The heart has an electric current running through it. The heart contracts and pumps blood throughout your body. This contraction is started off by an electric current, even though it is a weak one. This current begins in a part of the heart called the sino-atrial node, or the pacemaker, which sets the pace for the heart to beat. From the pacemaker this current follows a well-defined path through the rest of the heart. This movement can be recorded by electrodes, which are plastic plates placed on the chest and limbs to detect the current flow inside the heart. The graph recorded is the EKG and CKG, both painless tests. These tests detect disturbances in the pattern of electrical activity in the heart, called arrhythmia. They also check if any chamber of the heart is abnormally enlarged or if any of the walls have thickened. *(www.mmip.mcgill.ca/heart/egcyhome.html)*

ECHOCARDIOGRAPHY This painless ultrasound is an examination of the heart, used to evaluate structural conditions like the thickness of the walls; the way the heart walls move during exercise or rest; diagnose valve trouble; inflammation; congenital heart disease and congestive heart failure. Echocardiography uses high-frequency sound waves to produce images of the heart. A small transducer, like a microphone, passes over the chest, sending out impulses that bounce off the heart. The transducer records these echoes, and a computer converts them into a graphic display on the screen.

EXERCISE STRESS TESTING This is an exercise EKG electrocardiogram that's performed with controlled exercise such as a treadmill. The patient's maximum heart rate is calculated based on their sex and age, then the patient is connected to the EKG machine and exercises until the heart is beating steadily at the calculated rate. This test shows changes in the EKG pattern, especially for those with narrowing of the coronary arteries. If blood pressure drops during the test, this could be another sign of coronary artery disease. The stress test is also used for people who recently recovered from a heart attack, as an initial step in assessing the heart's blood supply. Please express any sensations experienced during testing (sometimes it's too much too soon). This test can detect coronary artery disease in 75% of cases.

NUCLEAR SCANNING This safe technique uses radioactive materials known as isotopes, to examine the heart. The isotopes used are harmless substances, and less radioactive than most x-rays. In nuclear scanning, the patient is given a small dose, either orally or injected. These isotopes flow through the blood system giving off radiation which is photographed by a special camera producing pictures of the heart. These pictures show how well the ventricles are working and where there is scarring, damaged or oxygen-starved areas of the heart.

● HOLTER MONITOR is a portable version of an EKG. It records the heart rhythm (pulse) during daily activities. This is worn for 24 hours or more. The heart waves are picked up by electrodes or patches placed on your chest. These waves are recorded on a tape inside the monitor. This recording is then scanned into a computer for analysis. Holter Monitors are used on patients who experience chest pain, dizziness, palpitations or fainting, most often caused by narrowing of arteries or heartbeat abnormalities. It may also show evidence of silent ischemia, which is like an angina attack (page 16) without chest pain. (See web: *www.bu.edu/cohis/cardvasc/testing/holter.htm*)

New Millennium Health Technology Provides Safer, Faster, Better Testing

DIGITAL TECHNOLOGY can take a routine test like a chest x-ray to a new height of quality and has many advantages. It's an environment saver because there are no film processing chemicals utilized; it is safer for the patient since it uses lower x-ray doses and reduces need for retakes and more exposure; it gives an instant picture and can be stored on a computer and transmitted instantaneously to the doctor's office, hospital or anywhere! *(www.ama-assn.org/insight/gen_hlth/rad/x_ray.htm)*

PET SCANNER: **Positron Emission Tomography**
is a unique 32-ring scanner that can detect and measure metabolic activity throughout the body and especially the brain. It pinpoints the source of cancers, neurological and heart diseases; thereby reducing all the expensive, unneeded operations, exploratory surgery and hospital stays! The PET scanner saves time, money and most important, precious lives! *(www.epub.org.br/cm/n01/pet/pet.htm)*

FOR SURGERY: XKNIFE STEROTACTIC RADIOSURGERY
uses a radionic *invisible blade* not a scalpel; this makes surgery non-invasive, bloodless, reduces complications, discomfort, hastens recovery. Excellent for brain tumors and arteriovenous malformations (AVMs). *(www.radionics.com)*

When needed, seek the highest quality, safest testing technology. Use these valuable guidelines as a source.

It's better to be safe than sorry. Medical and Hospital Emergency Centers do fast tests to relieve your mind to see if you have had a mild heart attack.

Dr. Paul Dudley White of Boston – Famous Heart Specialist's Wise Words

Dr. White, the former president of the American Heart Association, world famous pioneer heart specialist and our friend, gave this wise advice on taking care of the heart. We want to call your attention especially to the following points made by Dr. White in an article written for the American Heart Association. He begins with his startling facts that *middle age begins at 20*, and the *dangerous years are ages 20 to 40!* Here are Dr. White's words:

When does middle age begin? At 20, and it lasts until 80. And the dangerous years of this span are the first 20, not the last. These are the years when an overfed and under-exercised public is sowing the seeds of a coronary harvest.

I conceive the ages of man as five, Dr. White continues. *Birth to the 20th year; then a three stage middle age of 20 to 40, 40 to 60, 60 to 80; and finally old age – 80 to 100. The latter constitutes a steadily expanding horizon to which I see no eventual limit. Our life expectancy should keep rising indefinitely as research keeps making progress against disease.*

Unlimited Life Expectancy is Possible!

Dr. White stated, *The public can play an important role in this effort to push the life-span farther and farther. Physical-fitness and nutritional programs for men and women between the ages of 24 and 40 would guard against creeping degeneration and would instill lifelong good health habits.*

A man marries in his 20s; his wife cooks too much and too well – and between her cooking, the family car and the TV set, the man has gained maybe 20 to 30 pounds by the time he's 45. These are the years in which atherosclerosis (cholesterol blocking and clogging the arteries) and rusting of the arteries occur. This can ultimately reach the brain as a stroke, or the heart as a coronary thrombosis (massive blood clot). It may also affect the kidneys. This is why an apparently healthy man drops dead at 45 or 50. His death is not sudden at all; an unhealthy lifestyle has silently been building up for years!

Thank you – your explanation of the homocysteine theory of heart disease made this a red letter day in my life! – Dr. Paul Dudley White to Dr. Kilmer S. McCully, author *The Homocysteine Revolution.* (Page 153)

The automobile and the TV, I might add, should be the servants of the American public, not its masters. Despite the nation's generally unhealthy way of life, two factors work in favor of the American person, Dr. White concludes. *It is never too late – at any age – to begin controlling obesity and resuming a program of sensible exercise and a healthy diet. One excellent form, available to all, is walking. This should be brisk, and for a normally healthy person five miles weekly is not enough. Neither is one weekly 18-hole golf game.*

There you have it – from Dr. White, known as Dean of American Cardiology. Exercise and diet can be regular and enjoyable parts of the Healthy Lifestyle as you will discover by following this Bragg Heart Fitness Program we are outlining for you. *(www.openseason.com/st-agnes/whoispdw/default.html)*

Dr. Carrel's Eternal Life Successful Study

Dr. Alexis Carrel, eminent biologist and Nobel Laureate, of the Rockefeller Institute in New York City, *proved* to the world that *living flesh can be deathless!* In 1912, this Nobel Scientist took a sliver of a heart muscle from a chicken embryo and provided it with 2 essentials of life – simple protein food and correct drainage for the tissues. His simple laboratory experiment kept this tiny piece of embryo heart flesh tissues alive for 35 years.

This 35 year study proved that the heart tissue could have continued indefinitely! In 1912, Dr. Carrell received the Nobel Prize for this cell biology work. At the end of the experiment in 1947, this heart tissue had lived many average chicken lifetimes – the equivalent of hundreds of years of human life! It was called the *tissue of eternal youth.*

This amazing bit of embryo heart flesh doubled its size every 48 hours! Slices had to be cut away and discarded daily because its continued growth would have made it impossible to feed and cleanse the living heart cells. At the Rockefeller Institute, any scientist could observe *eternal life* before their very eyes! We can learn an important lesson from Dr. Carrel's revealing scientific demonstration with the tissues from a chicken heart. Namely, that if the body is correctly fed and its poisons and wastes are properly eliminated, life can continue indefinitely. *(nobel.sdsc.edu/medicine/laureates/1912/carrel-bio.html)*

Paul C. Bragg & Mentor – Bernarr Macfadden

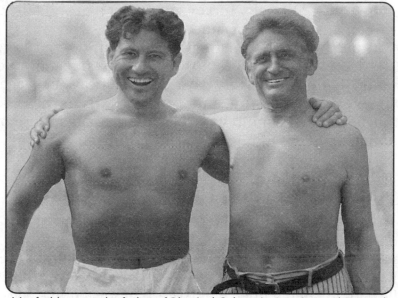

Macfadden was the father of Physical Culture in America and Bragg the father of the Health Movement and the originator of Health Food Stores. Paul C. Bragg began his life-time career in Natural Physical Fitness at the turn of the century by working with the famous Physical Culture pioneer, Bernarr Macfadden. Bragg was editor of Macfadden's Physical Culture Magazine, *the first publication to bring the basic principles of healthful living to popular attention in the U.S.A. They were credited with "getting women out of bloomers into shorts, and men into bathing trunks." Bragg started Macfadden's "Penny Kitchen Restaurants" during the big Depression Era, when they fed millions of hungry people for a penny each. Bragg helped develop America's first Health Spa at Dansville, New York, where this photo was taken. Bragg then opened Macfadden's Deauville Hotel, which gave undeveloped Miami Beach, Florida its great beginning.*

Macfadden – Founder of Physical Culture

My dad was associated with Bernarr Macfadden, who spent thousands of dollars to find the *oldest living humans* on earth. Dad was his main researcher on this project. This took my dad to many interesting, remote parts of the world, interviewing men and women from *103 to 154 years of age!* Dad found this work fascinating, because in his heart he always wanted to live a long life; not just the life of the average person which ends at about 70-72, but an active life that would last 120 to 150 years. His research proved it can be done! Now scientists worldwide are agreeing.

Zora Agha – Active at Age 154

In Constantinople, Turkey, my father met and talked with an amazing man named Zora Agha, who was 154 years old. What was this remarkable man doing at age 154? He was a baggage porter for the large railroad station. For 12 hours every day he carried heavy baggage! His eyesight, hearing and physical strength were unbelievable! His mind was keen and he had a sense of humor that kept him joking and smiling all day long.

Zora Agha's Secret of Youth – Healthy Natural Food and Hard Work (Exercise)

Through an interpreter, my dad questioned Zora Agha about the secrets of his astounding, long and healthy life. *His whole diet was simple* and uncomplicated. It included no refined or processed foods. Never in his life had he eaten refined white bread or sugar and – being a Moslem – he had never tasted any alcoholic drinks.

Dates Are Longevity Enhancers

When asked what his favorite food was, Zora replied readily, *dates*. The reputation of dates as a longevity enhancer has been verified by some of the other research on long-lived, healthy people. We discovered that people who eat dates have an abundance of vital energy, stamina and endurance. At one time, in the Atlas Mountains of North Africa, Dad was investigating a tribe of primitive Arabs who astonished him with their extraordinary strength and energy. He met men 70, 80 and 90 years old who were expert horsemen and could spend days in the African heat of 120° to 130°F without cause to worry.

But it was from Zora Agha in far-off Turkey that we first learned of the amazing value of dates as a healthful food. Dad also learned that he limited himself to 3 or 4 dates at a time. Zora knew the remarkable energy value of the *natural sugars found in dates*, but he also knew the body has only a limited capacity for handling these sugars, and so did his teeth. In the 154 years of his life he lost only 2 teeth! Dad was amazed when Mr. Agha displayed his teeth and gums. Every tooth in his mouth looked like a pearl – perfect, strong, white and hard.

Zora's Longevity Diet is the Biblical Diet

The vigorous 154 year-old Zora Agha also ate large amounts of garlic, one of humanity's *forgotten foods*. Garlic has been called *the poor man's penicillin* and as Nutritionists, we know its value in helping to keep the heart and arteries fit. (More on garlic and the heart later.)

Zora also said he ate only stale *black bread that had been dried in the sunshine.* He would purchase a loaf of black bread, slice it and let it dry in the sun. He never ate fresh bread. (Note: When traveling, we dry our health bread in the sun by putting it on the window sill. See, you can even have healthy, sun-dried bread when traveling.)

Other items of Zora's humble diet included ripe olives and lots of organic sun-dried dates, fruits and vegetables, greens and only occasionally lean meat and some eggs. He didn't use butter. The only oils he used for salads and cooking were olive oil and safflower oil.

These healthy, natural oils have been used in Turkey, throughout Asia Minor, and in the Holy Land, for hundreds of years. Zora's only beverage besides *water* was *mint tea*, which is the traditional beverage of all Arabs and Moslems. It occurred to my father that Zora Agha had naturally discovered the secrets of longevity. This was also the secret of the old Biblical Patriarchs who lived to fabulous ages and whose diet was so much like Zora Agha.

43

Harvard Says Eating Eggs May be Beneficial

Harvard University Medical School Researchers found that eating 2 to 3 eggs a week is unlikely to increase risk of heart disease. Plus, one egg has only 70 calories, is an excellent source of protein and essential nutrients including vitamins D, B-12, riboflavin and folate. (We prefer the fertile, free range eggs.)

Olive Oil Lowers Need for Blood Pressure Medication

Recent Massachusetts Medical Society Study shows that using extra virgin olive oil lowers the need for blood pressure medication. Participants in study ate a balanced diet, one half used extra virgin olive oil, the other half used sunflower oil, which had no effect on blood pressure. The ones who used the olive oil reduced their blood pressure medication by 50%! Eight of the 23 participants went off drugs completely! Systolic and diastolic pressure readings fell by 7 points, for those using extra virgin olive oil in their diet.

Olive oil enhances health by lowering "bad" cholesterol without affecting "good" HDL. Try Bragg's Organic Extra Virgin Olive Oil – tastes great and it's great for your health! (See web: www.oliveoilsource.com & bragg.com)

Life's Quantity and Quality
Depends Upon the Food We Eat

From this 154 year-old, healthy, energetic man we learned a great deal about keeping the heart fit by means of a simple natural foods diet and vigorous exercise.

Dad met only one Zora Agha in his lifetime. But we know that when the mass of civilized, humankind adopts a simple natural diet, there will be a lot of people who will reach Zora's remarkable age of 154 years.

Every intelligent person will agree that life's length and quality depends largely upon the food we eat. How carefully we select our foods will logically depend on how sound our heart, brain, nerves, body cells, tissues and vital organs will be tomorrow, next month, next year and 10 years from now. *The chemistry of the food a person eats becomes the chemistry of their body*.

Health, Happiness & Longevity – It's Up to You!

The results back up our teachings. You, and only you, can take proper care of your heart and body so that you may enjoy the *prime of your life* indefinitely! Most people reach their *prime* between 25 and 35, and then experience a decline. People who follow this Bragg Heart Program can attain the prime of life at any age and maintain and enjoy it for life! Now, plan and follow it!

If you have high or low blood pressure, you can restore it to normal by following the natural laws that keep your heart in good condition. My father's blood pressure always averaged 120 systolic over 70 diastolic, with a pulse rate in the 60s – just like a young man! We know that his case is not an isolated one – he's not a freak of perfect health. In our years of health consulting we have met countless men and women in almost unbelievably good physical condition at high calendar ages.

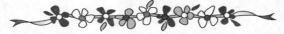

What you eat or drink or whatever you do – do it all to the glory of God and your human temple – I Cor. 10:30 and 3 John 2 are Bragg Crusades mottos.

Who is strong? He that can conquer his bad habits. – Ben Franklin

Chapter 5

Blood – Your River of Life

The body is composed of billions of tiny cells that are nourished by the blood carrying nutrients from the food we eat. As we read in the Bible, *The life of the flesh is in the blood (Leviticus 17:11).* If we can keep the blood in our bodies in perfect chemical balance – so that our vital organs and all the cells of our tissues are properly nourished – and if we keep the pipes of our bodies free from corrosion, there is no reason why we cannot enjoy a long lifetime of *youthful* living. Healthy blood and good circulation are the answers to a long, heart-healthy life free of premature debility and heart disease.

You can start to grasp the power you have to change your health by realizing that *all the red blood cells* in the bloodstream undergo a *complete change every 28 days.* They reproduce themselves about 12 times a year through a series of renewal processes that continue from the cradle to the grave. Our red blood cells are manufactured chiefly from the food we eat and the beverages we drink. If we put the correct nutrients into our bodies and keep our arteries, veins and capillaries clean, open and free from corrosion, we can increase our lifespan to 120 years or more, as expressed in Genesis 6:3 – *May your years be 120!!*

Your Bloodstream Carries Your Oxygen

Every one of the over 300 trillion cells in your body demands a continuous flow of life-giving oxygen in order to stay alive, do its job and remain healthy. Red blood cells carry this oxygen via a bloodstream teeming with life. Each of us has between 25 and 35 trillion red cells in our 5 to 6 quarts of blood - millions of cells in every drop!

We have so many of these red couriers of life and health that, in a normal healthy person, the death of 8 million red blood cells every second is not even felt! This is because, in the normal healthy person, 8 million new baby red blood cells are born into existence every second, ready to continue the work of transporting vital oxygen throughout the entire body.

Blessed are the pure of heart: for they shall see God. – Mathew 5:8

The Body's Main Nourishing Arteries & Veins – You Are A Walking, Talking Miracle!

Arteries

Veins

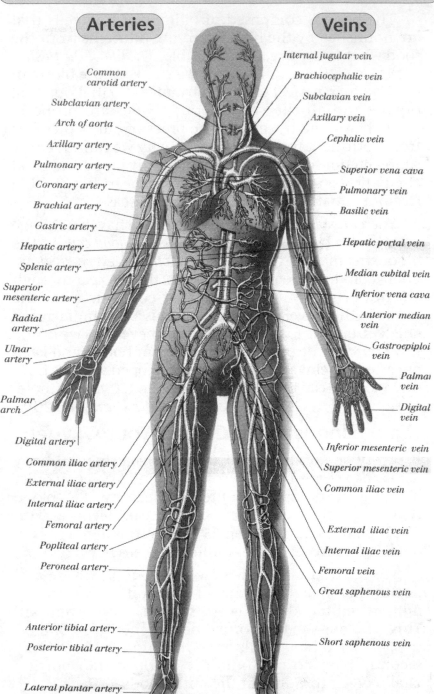

Common carotid artery

Subclavian artery

Arch of aorta

Axillary artery

Pulmonary artery

Coronary artery

Brachial artery

Gastric artery

Hepatic artery

Splenic artery

Superior mesenteric artery

Radial artery

Ulnar artery

Palmar arch

Digital artery

Common iliac artery

External iliac artery

Internal iliac artery

Femoral artery

Popliteal artery

Peroneal artery

Anterior tibial artery

Posterior tibial artery

Lateral plantar artery

Dorsal metatarsal artery

Internal jugular vein

Brachiocephalic vein

Subclavian vein

Axillary vein

Cephalic vein

Superior vena cava

Pulmonary vein

Basilic vein

Hepatic portal vein

Median cubital vein

Inferior vena cava

Anterior median vein

Gastroepiploi vein

Palma vein

Digital vein

Inferior mesenteric vein

Superior mesenteric vein

Common iliac vein

External iliac vein

Internal iliac vein

Femoral vein

Great saphenous vein

Short saphenous vein

Dorsal venous arch

Digital vein

46

Life Depends On Your Blood
Your River of Life

These red cell carriers of the body's oxygen are entrusted with the most important of life-sustaining jobs, but they can't circulate and distribute their cargo on their own. They are swept along in the bloodstream – the miracle river of life. The red cells and their non-oxygen carrying siblings, white blood cells, swim downstream together in the *plasma* of your bloodstream. Plasma is practically all water; it makes up over half the volume of blood. In addition to the blood cells, plasma carries food, antibodies (for fighting off threatening, foreign intruders), hormones (for regulating body systems) and platelets (for sealing vascular breaks and removing wastes). All the wonders of human life and health depend on blood, it's absolutely essential that you live a healthy lifestyle and keep your precious bloodstream unclogged, and healthy!

Teenagers Now Susceptible to Heart Disease

Nutritional biochemist, famous Dr. T. Colin Campbell of Cornell University has found that one out of two children born today will develop heart disease, and a new study from the American Heart Association Scientific Sessions (http://www.americanheart.org/), shows that heart disease actually begins developing early in childhood. Fatty deposits in the coronary arteries begin appearing by the age of 3, in children who partake in a typical American diet - processed foods laden with fats. By the age of 12, nearly 70% of our children have advanced fatty deposits, and by the age of 21, early stages of heart disease is evident in virtually all young adults! Dr. John Knowles, of the Rockefeller Foundation, has cited that 99% of all children are born healthy, yet are made sick as a result of their eating habits. The tender years of childhood should be the healthiest of all, bones are strong, hair is thick, liver and endocrine glands are functioning to full capacity, and they should have inexhaustible energy; yet, their bodies are being fed hamburgers full of steroids, antibiotics, hormones and chemicals; milk that is often indigestible which can cause ear aches, colds, allergies, asthma and lots of health problems.

The latest studies find "adult" diseases are related to what we eat throughout our early years in life. In fact, 95% of coronary disease can be prevented by implementing healthier eating habits earlier in life - reducing dietary fat and consuming more fresh vegetables, fruits and natural complex carbohydrates such as whole grains is very important.

Prevention is important - reward your child for good behavior with fresh fruits, instead of sugary processed candies; establish healthy eating habits before any damage to their health occurs.

Knowing these teachings will mean true life and good health for you.
– Proverbs 4:22

Childhood Obesity a Growing Problem

A recent shocking report in Newsweek Magazine, stated that one in three children that have long-term health problems are obese and the crisis is growing. The U.S. government estimates that 6 million or more of American children are now fat enough to endanger their health, with another 5 million on the threshold. Children today are 30% heavier than in 1990 due to extreme social forces, such as fast food and junk food TV commercials. The percentage of young people who are overweight has almost doubled in the past 20 years. Almost half of young people aged 12-21 and more than a third of all high school students don't participate in vigorous physical activity on a regular basis. Daily participation in physical education classes by high school students dropped from 42% in 1991 to 27% in 1997 and sadly might be even lower for 2001 and beyond.

High Fat, Sugared, Fast Junk Foods

Before 1988, about 6% or less of American children ages 6 through 17 were overweight. Since then, the number has jumped way up among children. So why is it that so many more children are overweight? The answer is painfully obvious, many children eat too much, especially the wrong foods and exercise too little. Children are driven to school or take busses instead of walking; they then come home and sit on the couch and watch ads for high fat foods on the television. A double whammy! The average American child spends from 15 to 24 hours each week watching TV, videos and the web – time that could be spent in physical activity.

If your food is refined, chemicalized and devitalized, or if its value has been diminished by wrong growing or cooking processes, you can starve to death on a full stomach because the important elements of nourishment have been removed.

48

Early Lifestyle Triggers Obesity

Lifestyle triggers obesity in kids. Many young people are not physically active on a regular basis and physical activity declines dramatically during adolescence. Regular physical activity in childhood and adolescence improves strength and endurance, helps build healthy bones and muscles, helps control weight, reduces anxiety and stress and increases self-esteem. It also helps normalize blood pressure and cholesterol levels.

There are numerous reasons for concern for these overweight children. Studies show that overweight children are at risk for many serious diseases such as high levels of blood pressure, insulin and cholesterol, making them excellent candidates for conditions like heart disease, diabetes and cancer. In addition, there is the emotional stress and depression associated with peer pressure and the stigmatism of being *fat*.

It's important to be supportive, accepting and loving of all children, overweight or not. A positive self-image is important for weight control. There are many ways to help an overweight child regain control of their weight. By cutting out 100 calories a day, he'll lose 15 pounds a year! Turn off the TV and video games and encourage physical activity; sports, handball, tae kwon do, rollerblading, swimming, trampolining, tennis, etc. Teach nutrition and healthy eating practices, not only by making healthy meals, but by example – eat the right foods and avoid fast foods, high sugar snacks, sodas and desserts altogether. Substitute healthy fresh fruit snacks and raw veggie stick snacks. Eat slowly and chew each mouthful thoroughly. Don't overeat. The Bragg Healthy Lifestyle establishes life-long healthy habits for all ages. Exercising, eating healthy foods and an occasional fast day helps teach children early to normalize their weight.

Every day the average heart beats 100,000 times and pumps about 1,800 gallons of blood for nourishing your body. In 70 years this adds up to more than 2.5 billion (faithful) heartbeats. Please be good to your heart and start this Bragg Healthy Heart Program for living a longer, happier, healthier life!
– Patricia Bragg, Health Crusader

Control Your Biological "Clock Of Life"

You can only get sound health from your healthy circulating blood nourished by correct food, liquids and air. These substances must be actively distributed throughout your body by the heart and blood vessels.

It is our contention that any person – regardless of age or physical condition – can rebuild themselves and have a stronger heart with cleaner *pipes*. My father demonstrated this with his own body. His abundant health, strength, endurance and stamina were the best proof of the success. He rebuilt his body from a hopeless, physical wreck into a sound, healthy and efficient cardiac machine with vigorous cardiovascular circulation.

Age is not a matter of how many years you have lived! It resolves itself into how clean your arteries are and the health condition of your blood. You can control your own biological *clock of life* . . . and there is no reason why you cannot fulfill the Biblical prophecy:

Man's days shall be 120 years. – Genesis 6:3

"Old Age" is Not Necessary

Do not be discouraged by your physical condition! *Remember that the body is self-repairing, self-healing and self-maintaining. Where there's life, there's hope!* Working with Mother Nature, you can start to rebuild a healthy bloodstream, and this will help you build a fit heart. To live long you must have a strong heart and clean blood vessels that are flexible, unclogged and elastic. *This Bragg Healthy Heart Fitness Program is your Blueprint to a New You with vital, fresh Super Health!*

Why grow old? *Old age* is not necessary – at least not as necessary as you may think. Instead of submissively growing old – *revolt! Grow young* – you can defy time! At 60 you can be bright-eyed as a bird and radiate the joy of living. At 70 you can be supple, youthful and full of sunny cheer. At 80 you can wear age like a jewel and who knows, you may become another Zora Agha!

Nine men in ten are suicides caused by their living habits. – Ben Franklin

Be your health captain and do what needs to be done.

You Can "Grow Younger" – It's Up to You

You stand at life's crossroads. Will you take the line of least resistance that often leads to a premature end, or will you, by disciplined living, climb to the clear heights of a healthful, youthful, radiant life? If you are going to strive for healthy longevity, begin today! Begin right now – don't procrastinate! Regard this Bragg Healthy Heart Fitness System also as a Program of Inspiration. It's intended to induce you to take stock of your life, get a fresh grip, and hoist yourself onto a higher plane so you can enjoy Health, Happiness and Longevity!

Why not *grow young?* If you have the desire, you will have the power, and by the Great Goddess of Health – Hygenia – you will succeed! Our Healthy Heart Fitness Program is going to show you how to create a powerful heart, a healthy balanced bloodstream and a strong circulatory system. We can't do it for you – You must!

We offer no *specifics* and no *cures*, for only Mother Nature and God has the power to heal a diseased heart! When you give your bloodstream the proper building materials, you can build a healthier and more fit body to help empower your body to heal you!

51

Healthy Benefits from Eating Onions and Garlic

Ancient Egyptians and Romans prized the extraordinary healing powers of garlic and onions. Recent research supports these claims. According to studies done by the nutrition department at Pennsylvania State University, consuming one medium onion a day may lower your cholesterol by 15 percent. The sulfur compounds in onions help lower dangerous levels of blood fats and help keep plague from adhering to artery walls.

Onions come in many varieties: yellow, red and white. Sweet onions like Vidalia, Maui and Walla Walla have a lower sulfur content than other more pungent varieties. To minimize tears, chill onions for half an hour before peeling and chopping. It's best to eat them raw for their full health benefit in salads, dips, spreads, soups, sandwichs and most foods. When cooking onions, lightly sauté them, for over-cooking can destroy important enzymes.

As for garlic's health role in protecting your heart, the cloves contain natural anticoagulants that help thin the blood, and they help protect against platelet stickiness – thus lowering the risk of clotting and even a stroke! Plus, garlic has potent immune-enhancing properties, it may eradicate many types of bacteria and fungi, including salmonella and candida; as well as inhibit gastrointestinal ulcers.

Remove garlic's outer papery skin. Let it sit for 10 minutes after chopping, to let the beneficial enzymes develop. Varieties of garlic and onions are: shallots, elephant garlic, garlic spears, leeks, chives and scallions – all beneficial to health!

The Highway to Higher Health and Happiness

Health and Happiness! To us, these seem inseparable. Our motto is: *To make my body a temple pure, wherein I live serene.* Promoting the welfare of our hearts and bodies is a loving, religious task. By *Health* we don't mean the everyday variety that consists of *not being sick.* We are referring to what we call the *Higher Health* – a sense of amazing well-being that makes a person proud to say with gusto, *I am feeling great today!*

We all agree that the chief aim of life is happiness! There is but one main avenue to happiness that we can recommend with confidence . . . and that is the Highway to Higher Health! Without balanced health – physically, mentally, spiritually and emotionally – it's difficult to have true happiness. The healthy ditchdigger is more in love with life than the sick, flabby millionaire. Good Health is the prime factor in attaining True Happiness. Keep your body healthy and fit and your mind and heart will rejoice in joy being a radiant health crusader!

52

Risk Factors of Angioplasty on Women

Women who undergo angioplasty are twice as likely to die than men are, stated researchers at the Montefiore Medical Center and Albert Einstein College of Medicine in New York. The findings were presented at the American College of Cardiology year 2000 conference. "This study is significant because we compared men and women for the same procedure, angioplasty, and for the same condition, heart attack. We found women to have 2.5 times the risk of dying during their hospitalization compared to men," said top cardiologist Dr. David L. Brown. The researchers looked at 1,044 patients, they found that women undergoing angioplasty for a heart attack are more severely ill and had more diabetes and hypertension than did the men.

Heart attack is the leading cause of death in women annually; angioplasty is generally considered to be the most effective treatment for heart attack. To prevent heart disease, be strong and start living The Bragg Healthy Lifestyle!

Recent studies revealed that fat stored in the body's "spare tire" around the waist increases risk for diabetes, heart disease and other serious health problems! Shocking fact: the bigger the waistline, the shorter the lifespan!

Herbs For Bone Strength and Healing Broken Bones

Wild Yam Root, Horsetail Herb, Oatstraw, Sarsparilla Root, White Oak Bark, Comfrey, Marshmallow, Alfalfa, Black Cohosh, Barley Grass, Plantain, Nettles, Goldenseal, Atnica Montatna, Dandelion, Sea Greens
– Linda Page, N.D., Ph.D., *Healthy Healing* (www.healthyhealing.com)

A Healthy Body and A Happy Mind

A happy and healthy body usually produces a happy, healthy mind. It by no means follows, however, that a happy mind will make a happy body. It would be glorious if the spirit could so triumph over the flesh. But alas the condition of the body usually has greater influence upon the mind, than the mind has upon the body. A person with a healthy sound body and who is spiritual, is seldom miserable, but it's rare for a sick, unhealthy person to be totally happy.

Latest research on a group of businessmen have found that those who had a spiritual connection – attended church or believed in a higher power – had fewer heart problems than those who had no spiritual connection!

3 John 2 is Our Bragg Motto For You
Dear Friend, I wish above all things that thou may prosper and be in health even as the soul prospers.

Studies have also found a strong correlation between personality traits and heart disease. The effects of stress on the heart is more prominent with those who were considered *Type-A* personalities – defined as competitive, aggressive, impatient, and sometimes hostile. Those with *Type-B* personalities are usually more relaxed and unhurried and had fewer heart disease problems. Most studies indicate the shocking facts that Type-A people are twice as likely to have coronary disease than Type-B people.

Healthy Fiber Habit: Have 3 to 5 teaspoons of raw oat bran a day in juices, soups, herbal teas, pep drinks, cereals, muffins, etc., plus eat fiber foods – organic fresh fruits, vegetables, legumes and whole grains! Fiber helps reduce blood cholesterol and the formation of varicose veins. Fiber helps keep you regular and reduces hemorrhoids. It's also a natural body-weight normalizer.

The heart propels blood through thousands of miles of blood vessels, pumping more than 30 times its weight in blood each minute. Even at rest, the heart pumps more that 1,800 gallons of blood a day. For all the work required of the heart, it is relatively small, about the size of a closed fist. In its pumping action, the heart delivers refreshed blood, filled with nutrients (from the food you have eaten) to the body's cells through approximately 60,000 miles of blood vessels, to maintain your health and well-being. (See pages 8 and 46.)

Every 33 seconds an American dies of heart disease. This year we will spend $287 billion for 60 million Americans (1 in 4) who have some form of heart disease.

Lifestyle Changes Help Remove Stress

Stress causes physical changes in the body that can increase the workload on your heart. During times of stress your body releases chemical transmitters that can cause changes in the circulation such as adrenaline and noradrenaline and several types of cortisone. Both adrenaline and noradrenaline have a direct effect on your heart, increasing heart rate and raising blood pressure!

By making positive lifestyle changes, such as deep breathing, prayer, meditation, stress-free walking and exercise, healthy diet and a positive attitude as you enjoy following The Bragg Healthy Lifestlye – this will help you can reap a longer, healthier, stress-free life!

AMA Says Legumes & Raw Nuts Improve Heart

A recent report from the American Heart Association's Conference on Cardiovascular Disease Epidemiology and Prevention, has found that eating beans and other legumes at least four times a week lowered heart disease incidence by 19%, compared to those who ate legumes less than once a week. There are cardiovascular health benefits for those who increase non-meat protein sources to their diet. Eating a diet rich in raw, salt-free nuts and beans improved blood lipid levels, in a clinical test of 25 to 74 year old participants.

54

Legumes are high-quality protein sources that are low in fat, high in dietary fiber and cholesterol free. In addition, legumes provide iron, folic acid, calcium, magnesium, potassium and B vitamins. Legumes have been consumed for more than 10,000 years and are a versatile, healthy food. The most common and popular legume is the soybean and other rich legumes include the blackeyed peas, chickpeas, lentils, black, red, white, navy and kidney beans. Just a cup of cooked dried beans as a source of protein, counts as meat in the meat group category of the Food Guide Pyramid. Legumes are also a healthy, delicious meat alternative in chili, pasta dishes, burritos, tostados, salads and blend to make delicious spreads and dips.

The dietary fiber found in beans has been shown over the years to decrease heart disease risks and help lower blood cholesterol levels by binding bile while decreasing intestinal transit time.

Study Shows There's Danger in Drinking Soda Pop

According to the Center for Science in the Public Interest, the average American teenager today is drinking twice as much soda pop as in 1974. One-fourth of all teenagers get 25% or more of their calories from soda, which is filled with sugar. In fact, teens consume two to three times as much sugar than the U.S. government guidelines recommend! The study linked increased soda consumption to heart disease, obesity, kidney stones and calcium deficiency.

Vegetarians have lower rates of heart disease and high blood pressure, colon cancer, osteoporosis, lung cancer, breast cancer, kidney stones, gallstones and diabetes, etc. – American Dietetic Association

Conrad Hilton Thanks Bragg for His Long Life!

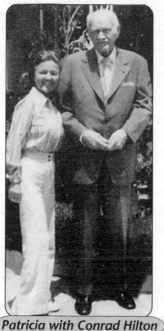

When the world's most famous hotel magnate, Conrad Hilton, was all of 80 and lying on his deathbed, we gave him a new lease on life by introducing him to The Bragg Healthy Lifestyle. He followed our instructions and discovered a whole new healthy, vibrant lifestyle! He was soon healthy, happy and fit, enjoying life! He even remarried at 88 years young! He remained active in business (half days at his L.A. office) to almost 100 years young! Mr. Hilton, at 88, was quoted in a *People Magazine* interview as saying, *I wouldn't be alive today if it wasn't for the Braggs and their Bragg Healthy Lifestyle!* Here's a photo of the grateful hotel founder with his healthy lifestyle teacher.

Patricia with Conrad Hilton

55

It's Never too Late to Learn and Improve

Men and women today are slowing down the ageing process by living healthier lives. The human structure is mechanically adapted for full energies and activities at 70, 80, 90 and older – clearly proven by the increased numbers of people worldwide who are healthy, hearty, clear of eye and keen of mind as they enter into their golden years. If you want to get the maximum joy out of life, start perfecting your human temple!

This is why we are Nutritional and Physical Fitness Crusaders. Happiness is largely dependent upon the care we give our bodies. Through the harmony of the flesh, we achieve the exultation of the spirit! Mental serenity is profoundly physical in its source. Through the purification of our body's living tissues we are helped to attain a balanced life of Supreme Health! Let's therefore put the health of our heart, body and soul first before everything, as everything else depends upon this!

Safer Minimally Invasive Surgery

Recent advances have now brought the open heart surgery technique to a viable safer alternative. Minimally Invasive Surgery was originally conceived by a Russian Surgeon in the early 1960's. The procedures are now performed through an incision less than ⅓ the size of a drastic full sternotomy (the former ranges from 9-12 cm long, the latter averages 30cm). Two types of procedures are being done using this technique: minimally invasive direct coronary artery bypass, or MIDCAB, and minimally invasive valve repair and replacement. MIDCAB is the "beating heart" surgery since the heart doesn't have to be stopped or placed on cardiopulmonary bypass (the heart-lung machine that oxygenates the blood and maintains blood pressure) and surgeons can operate while the heart continues to beat, which is safer for the patient. Due to the reduced incision size, this newer technique is less traumatic, has shorter recovery time and reduces the need for pain-killers. For more info see web www. heartsurgeons.com and http://picubook.net/absolute/MINIMAL.html

Follow This Heart Health Guide Faithfully

Would you trust the repair of your car to someone who had no knowledge of automobiles? Of course not! It is never too late to obtain and apply health knowledge. We have already described to you the structure and functioning of your heart and circulatory system and explained the importance of keeping the blood cholesterol at a low normal level. We suggest that you reread this book from time to time. Let this Program be your Faithful Guide on the Highway to Super Health.

The chemistry of the food a person eats becomes his own body chemistry. Perhaps the most valuable result of all education is the ability to make yourself do the thing you have to do, when it ought to be done, as it ought to be done, whether you like to do it or not.

Shocking Fact: 25% of hospital deaths are due to medical doctor errors. Play it safe – before any chemical drug treatments (chemo, etc.) or serious surgery, it's best to get 2 to 3 evaluations to be positive you are making the right decision for your future health! Once treatment or surgery is done, it is often too late to make amends, so the time to get consultation is before, not after the fact! It's your body and your right to help and judge in all decisions of your health and future well-being!

Chapter 6

The Discovery of Health

Health has sometimes been defined as *physical unconsciousness*. Not all physical unconsciousness is health, but the greatest compliment we can pay to the functioning of our body is to be unaware of it because it is running so smoothly. Most young people do not realize there is such a thing as health because when young, most have it in abundance.

With the passage of years, however, we tend to become aware, thus more *health-conscious*. The adage is so often true that says: *You spend your Health to gain your Wealth*. In later life, its reverse proves true: *You spend your Wealth to regain your Health*. The health-conscious person usually becomes so only after getting sick, and we are of the opinion that most people over 50 are a little sick. There would be no such thing as health if it were not for the lack of it. Most people begin to discover health's existence just when they need it the most. While *health consciousness* may be the result of impaired vitality, let us suggest this applies only to the common variety of health and *health consciousness*.

57

Invest in Your "Health Bank" for Comfort, Security and Happiness

Higher Health is essentially conscious or rather, it's *conscious of its unconsciousness*. It is *health pride – something you should truly cherish*. It's a will and a desire manifestation to live a long, happy, active and healthy life.

Can you think of any greater comfort, security and happiness than that of perpetual sound health? Or that any of your loved ones need never be stricken with an early death from heart disease? Or that no one need die at an early age, unless by an unfortunate accident?

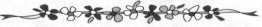

The unexamined life is not worth living. It is a time to re-evaluate your past as a guide for a bright future. – Socrates

Start Investing in Your Health Bank

Perhaps supreme super health seems *too good to be true*. Yet this ideal state of affairs is attainable by anyone willing to apply the principles of our Heart Fitness Program. It is our sincere conviction that the tragic prevalence of heart diseases, as well as many other diseases, is entirely unnecessary and is strictly within one's own control to prevent. Let health become a serious pursuit with you. The time and effort you spend following our Heart Fitness Program will be an investment in your *Health Bank*. This wise investment will bring you and your loved ones great returns in happiness and security. Always remember, *Your Health is Your True Wealth!* This teaching contained in our Heart Fitness Program – if followed faithfully and conscientiously – cannot fail to result in your acquiring and maintaining a more youthful, fit heart. Again, let us emphasize that our Heart Fitness Program does not offer a cure for heart disease, nor can it do anything until it is applied! But remember – the body can do miracles in healing itself if given a chance, as has been proven in thousands of cases.

The "Big Three" of Health and Longevity

Suppose you were told that you had to lug an unwieldy load of 20 to 50 pounds around with you wherever you went – walking, sitting, eating, sleeping – all day and all night. How would you feel about it? You would protest indignantly, wouldn't you? Yet that is exactly what you are doing when you are overweight! You are carrying around a load of unhealthy, flabby blubber. You are overtaxing all the functions of your body – especially your heart and circulatory system. Excess fat is dangerous! It exhausts the heart. Insurance statistics show that fat people are the shortest lived. Every pound of excess fat on your body shortens your life.

❤*Rule #1: Achieving and maintaining Normal Weight for a Healthy Heart.* Normal weight must be attained and maintained by a healthy diet, exercise and fasting. Forget drugs, they are dangerous!

Don't injure your system by over-feeding it and eating unhealthy foods.

❤ Rule #2: Daily Exercise for a Healthy Heart.

Vigorous daily exercise helps you to keep your weight normal, it will also stimulate a healthier flowing blood circulation throughout your body. It helps tone your muscles and vital organs, and aids all body functions, giving you the glow of Super Health!

❤ Rule #3: The most important is Proper Diet.

A healthy heart and body depends upon a clean, healthy bloodstream, and this depends upon the food you eat! We will discuss all of these points in detail later. When listing Proper Diet as point #3, we are saving the best for last. Your diet is the most important factor in controlling your ideal weight, nourishing your blood and protecting your heart from deadly-clogging cholesterol. Proper diet will strengthen you and make your heart a powerful *fountain of life* and a *fountain of eternal youth.*

Beware of Excess Body Fat

A normal amount of fatty tissue is an indication of health. But when fatty accumulations begin to bulge out here and there and destroy your youthful outlines – beware! These are danger signals warning you that it is time to take action to slim down your excess weight.

Excess weight invites heart attacks: It puts an undue strain on your heart and indicates you have been eating saturated fats that line your arteries with artery-clogging cholesterol. Excess fat is fatal to health, youth and makes you more prone to body injury, accident, disease and premature death! (Re-read bottom lines of page 3.)

The old myth that full cheeks and a plump body are indications of health still persists even in our so-called enlightened age. Disease gains a foothold more readily and is more difficult to dislodge when a person is overweight. Fat people have sluggish systems, less energy and endurance. Excess body fat indicates similar excess accumulations around the heart, kidneys and other vital organs, impairing their function.

The USA leads the world in heart disease, strokes, cancer and diabetes!

Don't injure your system by over-feeding it.
Over-eating will kill you long before your time! – Paul C. Bragg

Please Don't Be Overburdened With Fat

To be called fat or obese is an insult which reflects upon intelligence. What could be more unintelligent than allowing your body to be burdened with unhealthy and truly dangerous blubber? It's simply unwise and unhealthy to overstuff your body and burden your heart!

Fat people may be sluggish, tired or slow. Their vital resistance is sometimes low. If speed is necessary, some puff like a steam engine. Their heart and lungs are inefficient and have difficulty handling physical stress. Many fat people move with difficulty. Surplus weight lessens physical activity and often mental activity, too.

When an athlete is training for a contest, they eliminate all extra fat from their body. They know that fat lessens endurance and decreases physical energies. This also holds true in the military – maintaining normal weight is a must. A fat man often cannot fight well. Inefficiency and fat go hand-in-hand. They sleep and eat together – but they don't exercise together!

Your Waistline is Your Lifeline, Youthline, Dateline and Healthline

When you are fat you are flirting with old age! You are allowing the old age cells to gather in your body. When that happens you are playing with disease and should be prepared to pay the penalty.

Youthful body outlines must be maintained. This requires proper care of the priceless human *machine*. The rewards are well worth the effort! If you find fatty tissue accumulating, increase your exercise and reduce the quantity of food you eat and fast one day a week (see pages 155-161 for more on fasting). Don't be satisfied thinking that a naturally fatty surplus comes with advancing years! Beware if you make this mistake, for old age will arrive sooner coupled with serious illness and premature death.

The American diet is overloaded with too much food and the harmful fats that raise blood cholestrol levels and can cause fatal heart disease!

Studies prove: the bigger the waistline, the shorter the lifespan!

Keep Trim and Fit and Your Self-Esteem!

Always fight excess fat as you would your deadliest enemy! It often comes upon you like a thief in the night, silently and without warning. Sometimes you realize the danger only when serious difficulties are already staring you in the face. Then the fight is tougher, but fight you must! Your life may well depend upon your strength and faith!

An unshapely, obese body can destroy your health and self-esteem. You need to be proud of your body, not ashamed of your priceless, human temple. Self-esteem is as necessary to the spirit as healthful food is to the body. If you want to be efficient, eternally youthful, enthusiastic, full of the fire and fervor of life, *keep trim and fit and protect your self-esteem!* Build your body as an artist paints a picture or a sculptor molds a statue. Make your body an expression of the best there is within you! Let it reflect your very soul – your true self. Soon excess fat will find no lodging in your flesh!

What is "Normal Weight?"

There are numerous charts, tables and statistics on the subject of normal weight for particular ages, heights, etc. These are based on averages. However, *there is no such thing as an average person.* You may use such statistics as a general guide, but they should not be applied arbitrarily to determine your exact healthiest weight.

If you give your body the proper diet and ample exercise, you will naturally attain and maintain your best personal weight! To weigh a certain number of pounds does not necessarily indicate your proper measurement of waist, hips, etc. If you are firm and healthy – without excess fat – it doesn't matter whether you weigh more or less than the chart *average* for your years and height. The important thing is to find your own best weight as the result of proper care of your body. If your body is healthy, trim and fit, then your weight is normal for you. *Excess flabby fat is never normal!*

He who cannot find time for exercise, will have to find time for illness. – Derby

---

It's a lean, fit horse for the long, successful race of life! – Paul C. Bragg

FOOD FOR THOUGHT

Flexibility helps you feel young. Joints and ligaments lose their elasticity if they aren't stretched, then they grow shorter and tighter. Tension also settles into unstretched muscles, further sapping energy, making one feel older, less energetic and less inclined to get up and move around. The good news is that you can improve your flexibility at any age. The body is remarkably resilient, as long as you pay attention to your own comfort levels and be consistent. Some rejuvenating stretches can be found in yoga, ballet and basic sports stretches for all areas of the body. Remember to warm up before stretching to get the blood flowing. Jog in place and swing arms vigorously. Don't bounce when you stretch or hold your breath – gentle relaxed deep breathing is best. Be patient – don't push your body. While everyone can become more flexible, not everyone can be as limber as a dancer or gymnast. Challenge yourself, but don't push further than you can realistically go. You'll be amazed at the results. Be consistent – it's the key to progress. – UC Berkeley Wellness Letter
See web: *www.berkeleywellness.com*

62

Vitamin E is an antioxidant that helps prevent cardiovascular problems and enhances immune response. It is a primary defender against damaging free radicals. Stores of vitamin E decline with age, so it's important to add ample "E" rich foods to your diet such as: wheat germ, whole grains, raw nuts and seeds, beans, legumes, brown rice, cornmeal, oatmeal, sweet potatoes, green leafy vegetables and cold pressed vegetable oils. (See chart page 129)

Your birthday is the beginning of your own personal fresh new year. Your first birthday was a beginning, and each new birthday is a chance to begin again, to start over, to take a new grip on life. – Paul C. Bragg

The use of antioxidant supplements and a diet high in antioxidant foods has been shown to reduce cancer and heart disease and increase life expectancy. – U.S. News/Health Watch

Eating plenty of organic produce – fruits and vegetables – slows down ageing. The ageing that goes on under the skin, and chronic age-associated diseases, including heart disease, cancer and degenerative brain diseases can be slowed down, and even reversed in some cases with a change in diet. Adding lots of fruits, vegetables and garlic, taking vitamin and mineral supplements and avoiding saturated fats, can increase energy and add years to your life. Exercise is also important in delaying ageing. – Nanci Hellmich, USA Today

A teacher for the day can be a guiding light for a lifetime!
Bragg Books are silent health teachers – never tiring, ready night or day to help you help yourself to health! Our books are written with love and a deep desire to guide you to a healthy lifestyle. – Patricia Bragg

Chapter 7

Doctor Human Mind

A Sound Mind in a Sound Body

Shakespeare, almost 400 years ago, anticipated the dominant psychology of our time when he said, *It is the mind that makes a body rich.* It's true that the mind guides the body. Likewise, the body helps the mind and links us to the Infinite Spirit of Life! When we are truly healthy, we are brim full in body, mind and spirit. (3 John 2)

Our body relates us to the Universe in which we live – the Earth. We are related to Mother Earth through the food we eat, the water we drink, the air we breathe and the sun that warms us with its all-pervading power. All are essential for a healthy body and to the continuance of our life! All these nurturing things we need in as pure a form as Mother Nature and God have provided them, without depleting or denaturing them.

The food we eat is related to our health. Our bloodstream's system carries essential nutrients that provide the energy and vitality for the functioning of every part of the body. What we eat at this hour today will be nourishment in our cells within 24 hours.

If we eat organic foods as Mother Nature prepared it with her own unmatched chemistry – without losing essential elements – then it will meet our requirements for the growth, health and chemical balance of the body. It will build a powerful, long lasting heart for you. It will give you an alert and active mind. Healthy food will add life to your years – and years to your life!

63

Thy food shall be thy remedy. – Hippocrates

Beloved, I wish above all things that thou may prosper and be in health, even as thy soul prospers. – 3 John 2

Forgive and forget is the best advice for a healthy heart. Holding onto vengeful thoughts and grudges can increase your blood pressure, heart rate and muscle tension. Anger can actually thicken your blood and increase your risk for strokes and heart problems! – Natural Health

A fool thinks he needs no advice, but a wise man listens to others.– Proverbs 12:15

Correct Thinking is Important for Health

In the Book of Life, the Bible, Proverbs 23:7 tells us:
For as he thinketh in his heart, so is he.
When a sick person constantly convinces himself that he will never get well, it becomes almost certain that his negativity and troubles will carry him to the grave.

Flesh is dumb! We never want you to forget that statement. That is the reason we use it over and over again. The mind, your computer, is really the controlling factor in your entire makeup. Flesh cannot think for itself because only the mind does all the thinking. That is why you must cultivate Positive Thinking.

Your Mind Must Control Your Body!

The mind must have a will of iron and always be in command of the body. From this day forward learn how to substitute thoughts. When a negative thought – such as, *I am losing my energy because when you get older you start to lose energy* – enters your mind, replace it with positive thoughts that say, *Age cannot in any way affect my energy. Age is not toxic! I am ageless!*

64

Keep in mind always that whatever the mind tells the flesh, that is exactly what the flesh is going to believe and act upon. Your mind influences flesh. You must let your mind, make decisions for your body, because if your body rules your mind, you face a life of misery and slavery!

Are You Poisoning Your Body?

If you are eating the kind of food most Americans and people of other affluent industrialized countries eat, you are slowly poisoning yourself and dulling your brain. You are filling yourself with *foodless* foods and depriving your body of the natural nutrition it needs. You may also be among the many who hasten this suicidal process by adding toxic poisons such as tobacco, alcohol, coffee, tea and cola drinks.

There is a great deal of discussion in the media today about polluted air and water. What about a polluted bloodstream? Here is something you can do: Start today to detoxify your entire body and rebuild and revitalize it with healthy organic foods and healthy lifestyle living!

A Healthy Mind for Health and Long Life

What has your mind to do with health and long life? Far more than the majority of men and women realize! Think of your thoughts as powerful magnets, as entities which have the ability to attract or repel, according to the way they are used. A majority of people lean either to the positive or the negative side mentally. The positive phase is constructive and goes for success and positive achievements, while the negative side of life is destructive, leading to futility and failure. It's self-evident it's to our advantage to cultivate a positive healthy mental attitude. With patience, persistence and living The Bragg Healthy Lifestyle this can be accomplished.

There are many negative and destructive forms of thought which react in every cell in your body. The strongest is fear, and its child, worry – along with depression, anxiety, apprehension, jealousy, ill-will, envy, anger, resentment, vengefulness and self-pity. All of these negative thoughts bring tension to the body and mind, leading to waste of energy, enervation and also slow or rapid poisoning of the body. Rage, intense fear and shock are very violent and quickly intoxicate the whole system. Worry and other destructive emotions act slowly but, in the end, have the same destructive effect. Anger and intense fear stop digestive action, upset the kidneys and the colon causing total body upheaval (diarrhea or constipation, headaches, pains, fever, etc.).

Fear, worry and other destructive habits of thought muddle the mind! A crystal clear mind is needed to reason to your best advantage, enabling you to make sound, healthy decisions. An emotionally clouded mind often makes unwise and unhealthy decisions and might be unable to reach any positive conclusions at all!

What are the positive healthy mental forces or expressions? They are the ones that lead to peace of mind and inner relaxation, as opposed to the destructive habits which cause a tightening up of the entire system. This very second, let your mind take over your body.

A full stomach doesn't like to think. – Old German Proverb

A couple of generations ago, the only known main elements of food were the *proteins, fats and carbohydrates* – the primary building blocks and fuel supplies of the body. Since then, Nutritional Science has discovered that Mother Nature also provides many *various minerals, vitamins and nutrients* – which are equally essential for life and a healthy, harmonious functioning body. No one can be 100% healthy if this vital balance is disturbed, and yet it's constantly being tampered with by humanity. To give foods a longer *shelf life* in stores, certain elements are depleted and/or preservatives are added, thus changing the natural food content. These denatured foods, and even natural food, can become further devitalized by improper preparing, cooking, etc.

It's been said ***Americans are the most overfed and undernourished people in the world.*** And this is the main reason why the #1 Killer – Heart Disease – is having a field day in the United States! *Don't you be a victim!*

66

Drugs Control Addict's Mind!

The *drug addict* is the extreme example of the body ruling the mind! This is why the world is over-populated with drug addicts. The body's craving forces the mind to command the body to commit crimes of violence so that it may satisfy it with the drugs it craves. This is why the world is becoming crime riddled by drug addicts.

We maintain most of our bad habits simply because our minds are enslaved by our bodies. This applies also to alcohol, tea, coffee and other stimulants. The body rules by the false philosophy of *Eat, drink and be merry, for tomorrow we die*. This is false. You don't die tomorrow, but if you continue to live by this wrong philosophy, 5, 10, 20 years later you will be burdened with a sick, prematurely aged body tormenting you daily!

Bob Schuller's Hour of Power *Worldwide TV Sermon – Nov. 4, 2000 was based on Patricia's words of wisdom at the top of this page. You may see and hear this powerful message on the web: www.bragg.com*

Chapter 8

Doctor Deep Breathing

When You Breathe Deeply and Fully
You Live Healthier and Longer

When you pump a generous flow of oxygen into your body, every cell becomes more alive! This enables the four main *motors* of your body – the heart, lungs, liver and kidneys – to operate and perform better. Your miracle-working bloodstream purifies and cleanses every part of the body, including itself. This eliminates toxic wastes as Mother Nature planned, and fuel (food) and vital oxygen are carried to every cell in your body.

With ample oxygen your muscles, tendons and joints function more smoothly. Your skin becomes firmer and more resilient and your complexion clearer and glowing. You will radiate with greater health and well-being!

With the Bragg Super Power Breathing your brain becomes more alert and your nervous system functions better. You become free from tension and strain because you can easily take the stresses and pressures of daily living. Your emotions come under control. You feel joyous and exuberant. If negative emotions such as anger, hate, jealousy, greed or fear intrude, you can expel them by positive thinking and slow, concentrated deep breathing.

The deep breather enjoys more peace of mind, tranquility and serenity. In India, the great teachers practice deep, full breathing as the first essential step towards higher spiritual development. You can attain higher concentration in prayers and meditation by taking long, slow, deep breaths. Also, deep breathing stimulates your brain cells and promotes new brain cell growth.

67

Oxygen is the vital, precious, invisible staff of life. – Paul C. Bragg

On an average day your lungs move enough air in and out to fill a medium-sized room or blow up several thousand party balloons.

Super Deep Breathing Improves Brain Power

The person who breathes deeply and fully thinks more clearly and sharply. Oxygen stimulates your brain and logic and intelligence. The more deeply and fully you breathe, the greater your power of concentration and the more your creative mind asserts itself. You will also develop greater extrasensory perception within your body, especially the brain. Scientists at the Salk Institute for Biological Studies, La Jolla, CA, now know adults do generate new brain cells in the hippocampus, an area in the brain which is responsible for learning and memory. Deep breathing nourishes and fine-tunes the brain and entire body! *(www.salk.edu/NEWS/humneuro.html)*

Do read The Bragg Super Power Breathing book for it shows how to enjoy high energy vibration living! The more fully and deeply you breathe, the further you will travel to higher levels on the physical, mental and spiritual planes. Now close your eyes. Relax a few minutes while doing some slow, deep breathing! See web: *www.bragg.com* for some relaxing breathing techniques.

The Lungs Are Nature's Miracle Breathers

Every animal extracts oxygen from the environment in which it lives. Through their gills, fish extract oxygen from water. Insects get oxygen from the air through alveoli, or air cells, in individual openings set in segments of their bodies. Worms and other invertebrates breathe through the pores of their skin.

Vertebrate animals, including the human race, have those miracle mechanisms – the lungs. The mechanical equivalent would be a pair of bellows, though the lungs are far more intricate and adaptable. Human lungs are a miracle pair of conical-shaped organs composed of spongy, porous tissue. They occupy the thoracic cavity (chest) with the heart in the center, and are protected by the amazingly strong and resilient rib cage. The apex of each lung reaches just above the collar bone; the base extends to the waistline.

What makes up our lungs? About 800 million alveoli – air cells or sacs of elastic tissue – which can expand or contract like tiny balloons. If these little air sacs were flattened out and laid side by side, the flattened alveoli would cover an area of 100 square yards!

Tiny capillaries (blood vessels) thread the elastic lung walls of each of the millions of air sacs . . . and it is through these that the blood passes to discharge its load of poisonous carbon dioxide and absorb the vital, life-giving oxygen. The average person has five to six quarts of blood, which must be cleansed continually.

Air inhaled through the nose and mouth reaches the alveoli through an intricate system of tubes, beginning with the large trachea, or windpipe, which is kept rigid by rings of cartilage in its walls. The trachea extends through the neck into the chest, where it divides into two branches (bronchi), each leading into a lung cavity. Each bronchus divides into a number of successively smaller branches to bring air to every air sac.

You Have Lungs – Fill Them Up

Each lung sits perfectly enveloped in a protective elastic membrane, the pleura, whose inner layer is attached to the lung, and it's outer layer forms the lining of the thoracic cavity inside the rib cage. One end of each rib is attached to the spinal column, but the front of the rib cage is open. This allows the lungs to expand and contract. When you breathe deeply, filling every air sac, your thoracic cavity expands as your lungs fill with six to ten pints of air. This varies according to body build and size. Lungs occupy from 200 to over 300 cubic inches.

This marvelous breathing mechanism is yours for free! You are born with it. It functions without conscious effort, yet without it, you can't exist. Not even the latest inventions used by hospitals in emergencies, however ingenious, can equal the human breathing apparatus. Perhaps if human beings had to pay a fabulous price for their lungs and air, they would use them to full capacity all the time. Think of the big price you pay for only using them partially by shallow breathing. Remember, we are always only one breath away from death!. **Now, start enjoying slow, deep relaxed breathing and feel how your body responds.**

Shocking Sad Facts: Children and teenagers make up 90% of the new smokers in the United States and teenage and college smoking is on the rise! All tobacco should be banned – it's a killer to your lungs, heart and health!

The Importance of Clean Air to Health

It is essential to breathe clean air – air that's as free as possible from such chemicals as smog, car exhaust, natural gas appliance fumes and the many other toxic chemical pollutants. Also, our air needs to be as free as possible from mold, dust, dust mites and their fecal matter, animal dander and pollen. Everyone's health is helped in varying degrees by clean air. It is vitally important to live and work in an area which has clean air and which is free of all harmful fumes. It is also equally important to keep our homes pure, clean and free from dust, dust mites and debris! Most people cannot be truly 100% healthy and well until they breathe clean air, maintain a healthy diet and live a healthy lifestyle.

Pollutants Threaten the Lungs of All Life

Every living thing breathes. In the marvelous balance of Mother Nature, plants breathe in carbon dioxide through the pores in their leaves and give off vital oxygen – while animals inhale oxygen and exhale carbon dioxide. Both thrive in a healthy, natural balance.

Unfortunately, humans have played havoc with this natural balance by destroying forests and covering grass with pavement. They continue to poison our already over-burdened air with pollutants from motorized traffic and heavy industry. Wildlife, when it survives slaughter by humanity, suffocates in such polluted air. Fish die in polluted waters. How long can people survive in the midst of these environmental poisons which they continually create? This is a question of great concern to us. Read the classic book *Silent Spring* by our friend Rachel Carson, available in most libraries. If followed, her wise advice would have saved America and other nations billions of dollars and countless wildlife species! We desperately need more courageous and dedicated people like Rachel Carson to show the world the error of its poisonous killing ways!

*Breathing is the first place, not the last, one should look when
fatigue, disease or other evidence of disordered energy presents itself.*
– Dr. Sheldon Hendler, *The Oxygen Breakthrough*

Live Longer Breathing Clean Air Deeply

We advise those who have to live or work in smoggy, polluted cities to obtain a good air filter. We especially recommend filters which contain charcoal and a high efficiency particulate HEPA air filter. The charcoal removes most of the chemicals and the HEPA filter removes most of the particles. To be effective in an average room, the flow rate through the filter should be over 200 cubic feet of air per minute. The wise motorist will also install an air filter in his car for cleaning the air while driving in air-polluted cities. Auto stores and catalogs usually stock them.

When we are born, our lungs are new, fresh, clean, and rosy in color. If we could live in a pollutant and dust-free atmosphere breathing deeply all our lives, then our lungs would remain *as good as new* for a long life of use. Yet most people abuse their lungs! Some of this comes from external causes. The lungs and skin are the only organs of the body which are directly affected by external conditions, specifically, the air breathed into the lungs!

Mother Nature and God provide protection against a normal amount of dust contamination: tiny nose hairs serve as filters, and moist mucus in the passages leading to the lungs traps dust particles that we expel through the nose or mouth. The tonsils also serve as important guards to trap germs. The lungs protect themselves remarkably well by expelling carbon dioxide through oxygenation and by discharging toxins into the blood for elimination via the kidneys. *Your body is a miracle!*

Unfortunately, most civilized people today live in very unnatural conditions. Almost everywhere there are abnormal pollutants in the air we breathe, especially in urban areas. Our lungs are often overloaded with more contaminants than they can handle. These are passed into the bloodstream and to other parts of the body. Modern city dweller's lungs become brownish from car smog, soot, etc. Even in most farming areas, the lungs must contend with pollens, excessive dust, poisonous pesticides, fertilizers and other toxic chemicals. (Air purifiers and vitamin C helps.)

Shocking deadly fact: smog kills over 300 people yearly in #1 smog-riddled Los Angeles. This study has also estimated that this figure could triple soon!

Tobacco – Enemy of Your Heart and Health

Whether it's cigarettes, cigars or pipes, tobacco is one of the heart's worst enemies! Here is what Dr. Lester M. Morrison, noted California heart specialist and pioneer in the low-cholesterol diet for the treatment and the prevention of heart disease, said about tobacco:

Tobacco is a poison. Nicotine, the main ingredient of tobacco, is a poison affecting the brain, heart and other vital organs. The tobacco plant is directly related to the deadly nightshade family of plants. Aside from the chief poison, nicotine, there are other well-known poisons present in tobacco: arsenic and coal tar substances and carbon monoxide (when tobacco is burned).

Dr. Morrison also said, *Nicotine is the most noxious substance that affects the blood vessels in man. Nicotine is a powerful drug that constricts the arteries, narrowing still more the vital passageways of the blood, already clogged by other toxic residue. The tobacco smoker does double damage to his heart – first, by filling the bloodstream with the harsh poisons of tobacco and, second, by narrowing the arteries and other blood vessels, preventing a free flow of life-giving blood.*

Smoking Has Many Ways to Kill You!

The body has no defense against carbon monoxide produced by smoking. You have read about people committing suicide or being killed by carbon monoxide fumes. Why deliberately breathe them into your lungs? The coal tars in tobacco are the chief poisons responsible for cancer of the lungs, mouth and related areas of the body. It frightens us to think of what will happen in another 25 years because of the excessive use of tobacco. We are convinced that every smoker will eventually develop **lung, throat or some form of cancer** – if **heart disease** or something else doesn't kill them first!

The results of a recent federal health study found that cigars are no less hazardous than other forms of tobacco, and therefore needs stronger federal regulation! The absence of such warning labels on cigars could lead consumers to erroneously conclude that cigars don't carry health risks. Beware – there is no safe form of deadly tobacco! Cigars are becoming tremendously popular and sales have jumped 18% recently. Yet cigar smokers and tobacco chewers face grave risk of diseases such as mouth, throat, esophageal, larynx and lung cancer, as well as coronary heart disease and chronic obstructive pulmonary disease. Fact: cigars contain up to 90 times as much of some cancer-causing agents as cigarettes do!

Emphysema Smothers it's Victim

Emphysema, another killer disease from smoking, is on the rise. Recent medical reports show that as many as half of all American men are suffering from some degree of emphysema. In this disease, the tars, nicotine and other destructive poisons of tobacco lodge in the lungs' small air sacs, causing the sac walls to become very thin or to break down entirely. Soon the blood is no longer able to exchange poisonous carbon dioxide for life-giving oxygen. This self-destructing victim dies of oxygen starvation – being slowly smothered to death from within.

Emphysema is not a quick killer. It creeps up slowly, first with a slight cough – especially on arising. Then it attacks the smoker day and night. Slowly, air sacs are almost completely destroyed. The victim doesn't die suddenly, but lingers on steadily deteriorating. They are forced to stay near an oxygen tank because the disease is shutting off their oxygen. When the lungs can't operate any longer even with pure oxygen, the victim then dies.

Our breath is our life! We can live days without water and weeks without food, but only minutes without air. It's the oxygen in the air we breathe that's the greatest purifying force in Mother Nature! To get this oxygen into the lungs and bloodstream, we must breathe it in!

Smoking tobacco is against every Natural Law. When you attempt to break a Law of Mother Nature, it will break you! *The heart needs large amounts of oxygen to function.* Any disease that diminishes oxygen is going to destroy the health of your heart, lungs and entire body.

Most heavy smokers are snorers and are at 1.7 times greater risk of heart disease than silent sleepers and at 2.08 times greater risk of stroke and heart disease combined. – Finnish Medical Study

---

Cigarette smokers have 50% higher atherosclerosis and hypertension deaths!

Vitamin C Protects Heart, Arteries & Body

Vitamin C is one of Mother Nature's most essential elements for good health. In addition to its other vital functions – such as prevention of scurvy, vitamin C is also active in preventing capillaries hemorrhaging, those tiny blood vessels that directly feed the body's cells. (We take 1,000 to 3,000 mg mixed "C" daily, plus grapeseed extract.)

Smoking Robs Your Body of Vitamin C

Tobacco neutralizes Vitamin C in your body, robbing you of its vital protection. Dr. W. J. McCormick – Canada's "C" Specialist – found in lab and clinical tests that *the smoking of a single cigarette robs the body of the amount of vitamin C contained in 1 medium sized orange.* A *pack a day* smoker would have to eat 20 oranges for enough "C" in his body! Tobacco is not the only "C" thief, polluted air and foods with preservatives are also.

When capillaries in the artery walls hemorrhage, there is additional blockage to the blood flow. When this occurs in the heart or brain, a serious clot may form. In the legs and feet serious breakdown of the capillaries may occur. Sometimes this leads to gangrene, requiring an amputation and sometimes it causes varicose veins. So you can see how essential Vitamin C is to the healthy functioning of your heart, bloodstream and entire body.

All Smokers – Stop Smoking Today!

Many smokers are so addicted to this unhealthy and filthy habit that they become cry babies, saying, *It's impossible for me to break the habit of smoking.* All we can say is, Rubbish! *Who controls your body – the tobacco or you?* Flesh is dumb! It has no intelligence. Your mind (your miracle computer) must control your body! The mind can always force the body to obey its orders!

> *QUIT SMOKING! All smokers must stop this vicious, deadly habit that destroys health, youth, energy and life.*

Caffeine is a Dangerous Habit: How much coffee do you drink?
Research found that 17% of Americans have 1 cup daily, 15% – 2 cups, 10% – 3 cups, 7% – 4 cups, 12% – 5 or more cups and 38% no coffee at all.
Never use coffee and caffeine products if you want super health!

DEADLY SMOKING FACTS!

✝ Tobacco use and second-hand smoke will eventually kill 1/5 of the developed world population: about 250 million people.

✝ Of the 50 million Americans who smoke, one third to one half will die from a smoke-related disease. All will reduce their life expectancy by an average of nine years.

✝ Smoking acts as either a stimulant or a depressant, depending upon the smoker's emotional state.

✝ The average pack-a-day smoker takes about 70,000 *hits* of nicotine each year and with 2 packs it's 140,000 *hits*.

✝ "Second hand smoke" hurts non-smokers: it speeds up the heart rate, raises blood pressure and doubles the amount of deadly carbon monoxide in their blood.

✝ Secondary smoke contains more nicotine, tar and cadmium (leading to hypertension, bronchitis and emphysema) than mainstream smoke.

✝ Babies born to mothers who smoke tend to have lower body weight and smaller lungs.

✝ Lung illnesses are twice as common in smokers' children.

✝ Children and teenagers make up 90% of the new smokers in the United States – and teenage smoking is on the rise!

✝ The death rate from breast cancer ranges from 25% to 75% higher among women who smoke.

✝ Female smokers may face a higher risk of lung cancer – as much as twice the risk of male smokers, according to Dr. Harvey Risch's study at Yale University.

✝ Your body contains over 60,000 miles of blood vessels. Smoking constricts those vessels, depriving your body of the important fresh, rich oxygen it needs.

✝ Tobacco is the main introduction to more deadly drugs.

✝ Teens who smoke are far more likely to engage in other risky and life-threatening behaviors than non-smoking teens (including using other dangerous drugs, violence, gang involvement, carrying weapons, and engaging in premarital sex, which often results in pregnancy or disease).

✝ Cataracts, cancer, angina, arteriosclerosis, osteoporosis, chronic bronchitis, high blood pressure, impotence, diabetes and respiratory ailments are linked to smoking.

75

A Deep Desire Has Great Power

In our Bragg Health Crusades worldwide we have had health *students in our classes who have smoked for as many as 50 years – and they stopped, without tapering off.* They simply made up their minds to stop smoking at once – and they did. They stopped without the use of nicotine patches, nicotine gum, etc., as these are dangerous, too!

Of course the brave souls who are quitting suffer for a few days as their nerves cry out for the nicotine *fix* of the deadly tobacco. However, they find the intestinal fortitude and purpose to take the brief punishment of their withdrawal discomforts. They are fighting a monster that controlled them. They can and will win their battle!

To be effective in changing a bad habit into a good one, rational thought must be accompanied by deep feeling and desire. If you desire a Healthy Heart strongly enough, you can and will conquer the tobacco habit!

Picture yourself as you would like to be. Believe for the moment that such an image is possible. In forming good habits and breaking bad ones, we have to deal with *thought habits. As a man thinketh in his heart, so is he.* Think, *No smoking!* Tell yourself over and over that your smoking is slowly killing you and that it's your enemy. Say to yourself over and over again, *Tobacco in any form is a killer and I am through with this vicious poison forever!* Repeat, *I will not smoke!* over and over again. You will soon become master of your body instead of a slave to the tobacco habit!

Be Your Body's Health Captain

You must not be a slave to any bad habits that will damage your heart or body and contribute to a heart attack. That goes not only for tobacco, but for coffee, tea, caffeine, drugs, alcohol, salt and saturated fats. *Free yourself from the bondage of these killing habits!* Look at these poisons as your heart's enemies. For a strong, healthy heart you must faithfully practice *Health Mindedness.* In your mind's eye see yourself as you wish to be – strong, healthy and youthful. A person who is in charge of his body is not a slave to unhealthy lifestyle habits!

Say to Yourself: If it is to be – It is up to me!

- ❤ "I will not use tobacco."   ❤ "I will not use salt."
- ❤ "I will not drink coffee."   ❤ "I will not over-eat."
- ❤ "I will not drink black tea." ❤ "I will not drink sodas."
- ❤ "I will not clog my arteries with saturated fats."
- ❤ "I will not drink alcoholic drinks."

Habits that destroy the health of your body must be broken with a strong willpower! Say to yourself repeatedly and believe it, that your intelligent mind will health captain your body towards super health! Let no person or circumstances break your iron willpower! Let no one brainwash you! You must do your own thinking! You can and will control your own mind, body and health. With inner strength you break bad habits of all kinds!

Coffee and Non-Herbal Tea are Drugs

Coffee is a harmful stimulant to the heart. It contains the drug caffeine which makes the heart beat faster and puts it under an undue, unhealthy strain. Coffee also contains tars and acids which are injurious to the heart, blood vessels and other tissues. These same agents are also present in de-caffeinated coffee. Don't drink coffee – it has no nutrients and no vitamins or minerals! Coffee is worthless and harmful to your health! The same goes for non-herbal tea. Don't contaminate your bloodstream with these toxic substances – tea contains tannic acid!

Study Shows Cola Drinks Toxic To Body

What do cola drinks contain? Three toxic stimulants and carbonated water! Colas contain caffeine, phosphoric acid and refined white sugar (also some diet colas contain toxic aspartame); all are toxic *empty calories* without any health nutrient value. They also contain carbonated water, which irritates the kidneys and the liver! Recent study says: *Don't drink colas or any sodas – and don't let your children ruin their health with these drinks!*

Life is learning which rules to obey and which rules not to obey and the wisdom to tell the difference between the two.

Alcohol is a Depressant and Killer!

Alcohol, generally considered a stimulant, is actually a depressant. It dilates the blood vessels, in time breaking the tiny capillaries, especially of the nose, cheeks, neck and ankles (example: red, swollen nose of hard drinkers). Alcohol is also a relaxant and dulls and paralyses the brain. The drinker loses good judgement and control of the body, and is therefore the cause of thousands of car accidents, crimes, killings, rapes and unnecessary deaths. *Drinking alcohol is dangerous and an unhealthy way to relax!*

The chief toxic effect of alcohol is on the brain and nervous system. Alcohol *burns up* by depleting the body of vitamin C and also B (the essential nerve vitamin). This, in combination with capillary dilation, can lead to brain hemorrhaging – which in turn, can lead to paralysis. Medical research has shown that the boisterous actions, loud speech, joviality, bravado and *devil-may-care* attitude of the alcoholic are actually the beginning paralysis of certain parts of the brain!

Stay away from alcohol! It is nothing but *empty calories*. It will burden your body with unhealthy, flabby fat, in addition to its other toxic, poisonous and injurious effects. The *numbing effect of alcohol* on the pain centers of the brain and nervous system is a *special danger to anyone with a heart condition*. Without Mother Nature's warning signal – pain – a heart attack, which might have been averted, may prove fatal.

No Self-Drugging!

If you try to prescribe drugs for yourself, the side effects and long-term results could be serious! Even though constant TV ads keep telling us what to take to solve aches, pains, upset stomachs, insomnia, etc. It's wise to seek advice from your alternative health care advisor and then follow the directions exactly!

The alcohol habit is most harmful and must be eliminated!

Coffee increases free fatty acid levels in the blood and causes degenerative diseases! "There is a strong likelihood that caffeine may prove to be one of the most dangerous mutagens to human life." – Cancer Research

Chapter 9

Doctor Exercise

Mind Over Muscle

The saying, *If you don't use it, you lose it,* certainly applies to the 640 muscles of the human body. When you don't exercise regularly, your muscles lose their firm, supple tone. Over time they become soft and flabby.

If overweight, make up your mind that you want to trim down to your normal weight. This is more difficult than it seems, because the mind has a way of making excuses for an overweight body. For instance, you may say to yourself, *It's normal for me to be fat. I'm the plump type,* or, *I eat so little, yet I remain fat.* The latter may be true – but remember it is what you eat – not how much! And it is never normal to be obese!

Your mind must control your body! Flesh is dumb and flesh is weak. Flesh often demands fatty, starchy, sugary foods. Either your mind rules the body or the body rules the mind. Be positive! Tell your body that your mind is going to be the best health captain!

79

Exercise Daily for a Powerful Heart

Remember that it is a lean horse that finishes the long race! If you want a long, healthy life, keep your body trim and fit. Once you have trimmed down to your normal weight through proper diet and daily exercise, there will be a huge difference in the way you will feel! You will be bubbling over with vitality and energy. You will be unafraid of life's challenges and free from the fear of heart trouble and other illness!

Laziness is a vicious habit. Sitting too much can ruin your health and is a bad habit. You need to devote *1 to 2 hours every day* to some kind of vigorous exercise. The simplest and best is brisk walking for a strong heart – preferably up and down hills, or walking up and down steps.

The surest way to fail is to determine not to succeed. – Sheridan

Duty is a matter of the mind. Dedication is a matter of the heart.

Enjoy Exercising – It's Healthy and Fun!

There is great hiking near where we had a home in Hollywood, California, where Mt. Hollywood rises some 2,000 feet in famous Griffith Park. We enjoyed early morning hikes up the mountain to greet the sun rising and then run down. Also, in Santa Barbara, we always enjoy ocean swimming and hiking the surrounding hills.

We love to walk, jog and climb mountains. We take time to walk or jog daily, or we swim, play tennis or ride our bikes. We work out 3 times a week with a progressive weight training program, which helps keep our bones and muscles healthier and stronger. See pages 97 to 99.

Exercise is the greatest single factor available to us for removing any blockages and unclogging the arteries and blood vessels, and for increasing the vital flow of oxygen-enriched blood throughout the heart and body. Recent studies show that exercise can reduce the risk of developing adult-onset diabetes as well as breast cancer. The famous Harvard School of Public Health Researchers (www.health.harvard.edu/fhg) studied a group of 70,000 women. Results: 46% lowered their risk of diabetes with daily vigorous exercising and brisk walking.

The Miracle Life of Ageless Jack LaLanne

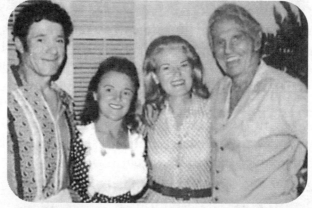

Jack LaLanne, Patricia Bragg, Elaine LaLanne & Paul C. Bragg

Jack says he would have been dead by 16 if he hadn't attended The Bragg Crusade. Jack says, *Bragg saved my life at age 15, when I attended the Bragg Health and Fitness Crusade in Oakland, California.* From that day, Jack has continued to live The Bragg Healthy Lifestyle, inspiring millions to health, fitness and a long fulfilled, happy life!

Develop Strength from the Inside Out, Not from the Outside In

Remember that from the day you were born into this world, to the day you die, your 640 muscles play an important role in everything you do. Think of it – *more than half your body is sheer muscle!*

It isn't the muscles that you see that count as much as those you don't see! Along the 30-foot gastrointestinal tract there are muscles to force food along this tube. The work of bringing adequate amounts of air into your powerful lungs also requires other strong muscles.

And above all, *the greatest muscle* in your body is *your heart, your number one pump.* It is the heart that pumps the blood supply into the body's 640 muscles. And the more we bring these 640 muscles into play, the better our heart, circulation, physical condition and our entire state of health will be! You have four more extra *pumps* that can also help this whole process – they are your two arms and your two legs – use and exercise them!

Brisk Power Walking is the King of Exercise

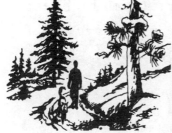 Brisk power walking is the best form of aerobic exercise because it brings most of the body into action which helps open up blocked blood vessels and builds your endurance. Your heart grows in strength and efficiency, able to function with less strain. Also, many problems and upsets get solved on walks. As you walk, grasp yourself in the small of the back and feel how your entire frame responds to every stride. Feel how your chief muscles are functioning rhythmically. No other exercise gives the same harmony of coordinating sinews and the same perfect circulation of the blood. Brisk power walking is ideal for you, your health and your heart! (We also enjoy ocean swimming.)

The goal of exercise and weight loss should be to reduce abdominal deposits of fat that lowers the potential for cardiovascular disease (page 60).

Faith can place a candle in the darkest night.

Walk 2 to 3 Miles Daily – It Does Miracles!

You should try to walk 2 to 3 miles daily, and some times try doubling it. Don't give yourself excuses. *Make a daily walk a permanent part of your Bragg Healthy Heart Fitness Program* – all year and in all climates. Conrad Hilton walked in the sun and rain and loved it. Regardless of what other exercise you do, your daily walk is a *must*!

Of course, you may take it in the form of golf if you enjoy this social sport. But it's best not to ride around the golf course in an electric cart! This makes a farce of the whole thing. Walking is what your heart needs. We are inclined to agree with Mark Twain, who said, *Golf is a good way to spoil a good walk.* But, if it takes the game to make you walk, do so. The result is almost the same – healthily functioning muscles and quickened blood circulation, plus a sense of harmony and happiness.

Although the outdoors is preferable – where you can get the most fresh air – indoor walking is far better than none at all. In winter, you can try hallways, porches or shopping malls. When on health crusades around the world, we take an evening brisk walk through the corridors, and up and down the stairs of our hotel. If a roof terrace is available, we prefer this open-air space.

Expert Advice on How to Exercise

Often you may ask yourself, "Why aren't you closing in on your ideal weight?" You're trying to workout and exercise, but it doesn't seem your bathroom scale is showing you any results - your weight appears the same as when you started out. Here are some tips from the exercise experts:

● An effective weekly exercise program to get your heart in shape should include one rigorous program that makes you sweat; two moderate exercise programs, and one easy session. For example: taking an aerobics class, or a run and after a more relaxing yoga or stretching class.

● In the initial phases of exercise training, you may get a post-workout drop in blood sugar that causes cravings for simple carbohydrates like sweets. However, the cravings should disappear a few weeks into your exercise training. Have delicious fresh fruits handy such as organic apples, oranges, pears and bananas, rather than reaching for an unhealthy chocolate bar.

● Drink at least 64 ounces of purified (distilled or reverse osmosis) water daily (8 glasses). Drinking water has a huge effect on exercise. Dehydrated exercisers worked out 25% less than those who drank water before and during workouts.

To Enjoy Your Daily Walk Is Important

Your walking should never be done self-consciously, no heel and toe routine and no time limiting. Let it be the most functional and enjoyable of exercises. Walk naturally – with head high, spine stretched up, chest out and tummy in. Swing your hips, arms and body into action. Walk as though your legs began at the middle of your torso. Breathe deeply! You will feel physical elation and will carry yourself proudly with body erect and arms swinging easily from your shoulders.

Move at your own pace, with a free spirit and a light heart. If you want, listen to motivational tapes or music. As you walk, your body ceases to matter, you become as near a poet and nature philosopher as you will ever be.

Walk your worries away! As blood courses through your arteries, cleansing and nourishing your body, you are filled with a sense of well-being that clears your mind of troubles and nourishes it with positive thoughts. As we stride along on our hike, we say to ourselves and sometimes aloud with each step – *Health! Strength! Youth! Vitality! Love! for Eternity!*

It's beneficial to also take a hiking tour once a year. Select interesting areas which you, your family and friends would like to see, and hike about 15 miles daily. You will broaden your knowledge of our beautiful planet and of Mother Nature, as well as help to build a more powerful, healthier and long-lasting heart. The websites listed below will help you in your selection.

Walking-Running – Perfect Conditioners

We love jogging and walking – because a *run a day helps keep heart attacks away!* We also enjoy light jogging, as practiced by athletes in training workouts. Do this with an easy sustained pace, head up, shoulders back, arms swinging naturally. All athletes and trainers worldwide consider running and jogging as perfect conditioners.

Websites to inspire you into healthy walking, jogging and hiking programs in your area:

- www.fitnesslink.com/mind/aware.shtml • www.sierraclub.com
- www.fitconnection.com/ • www.activevideos.com/walking.htm
- www.outdoorsclub.org/index1.htm • www.gorp.com/gorp/activity/hiking.htm

Enjoy Exercise & Jogs for Longer Life

On our world Bragg Health Crusades the first question we ask the hotel manager is, *Where is the nearest park where we can take our daily exercise?* And off we go sometime during the day. We prefer to go early in the morning or late in the afternoon. Each person, however, should choose the time best suited and available to them.

We are so pleased to find that all over the world today running and jogging have become an accepted method in the pursuit of Heart Fitness by people of all age groups. Many cities have hiking and jogging clubs, which anyone may join. We have had the pleasure of running with folks around the world; including Europe, England, Australia, New Zealand, Asia and throughout the U.S.

It is universally accepted that exercise is important for the promotion of physical, mental and emotional health. A daily run or jog – when adapted to the individual's physical condition and age – will improve endurance, produce a sense of well-being and help to maintain total body fitness (plus each step gives your body a little massage, trampolining does also). Exercise helps increase resistance to sickness and disease, and helps make the heart stronger and life longer!

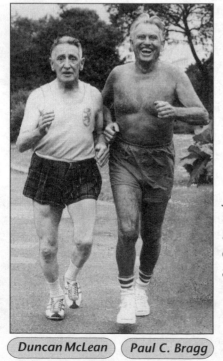

Before starting on your exercise program, it's wise to seek advice from your health practitioner. Also, be sure that you choose a soft surface to run or jog on, such as grass or sand. Jogging on hard surfaces, such as concrete and asphalt, could accumulate damage to knees, hips, ankles and organs.

❦❧❦❧❦

Bragg with friend Duncan McLean, England's oldest Champion Sprinter, (83 years young) on a training run in London's beautiful Regent's Park.

Duncan McLean   Paul C. Bragg

84

Exercise is the Best Fitness Conditioner

A daily program of walking, running or jogging is a quick, sure and inexpensive fitness conditioner. Be faithful to your exercise routine for true heart fitness. Women will be especially pleased when they see fat change to lean, as the inches fly off their waistlines and hiplines – all the while improving their health! Men and women, both please remember your waistline is your lifeline and also your dateline! A person with a trim and fit figure always looks more youthful and attractive!

If you are a *softie* and feel you cannot get outside for your run or jog on cold and rainy days – stationary inside jogging to music or your favorite talk show will work too. Stay in one place and lift one foot at a time about 6-8 inches from floor – it's best to start easy and gradually build up to faster, longer periods. Remember to exercise where you get the most fresh air – on the patio, front porch, or inside or outside rest areas at work.

Heart Disease & Irritability & Dominance

New studies from the John Hopkins School of Medicine and the University of Maryland have found that irritability and dominance may cause coronary heart disease. *Until recently, most research centered on the role of psychosocial factors*, says Dr. Aron Wolfe Siegman. The study involved 101 men and 95 women, the average age was 55 years. The research found that a full-blown outward expression of anger is a risk factor for coronary heart disease in men, and for women – subtle, indirect expressions of antagonism are big risk factors. Also, expressions of irritability with anger are risk factors for coronary heart disease. (See web: *www.sinatramd.com*)

Death rates from heart disease are up 4 to 7 times higher among people with hostile, mean attitudes, stated by Dr. Redford Williams, Duke University Medical Center.
www.mcis.duke.edu/cgi-fps/getPerson.pl?personid=2129

Love is living in harmony with all those around
you and all that surrounds you. – Amrit Desai

Only 20% of American's have some form of regular exercise! This is causing poor health and more cardiovascular disease! Regular exercise is important for your Bragg Healthy Heart Program. Please start your exercise program today.

Exercising in the Sky – You Arrive Healthier

We even get our jogging in while thousands of feet high in the air, soaring the skies in a airplane. We just go to the rear of the plane and jog and stretch. We never arrive stiff and tired. Learn to take advantage of any spare moments for stationary jogging during the day, whether you are an office worker, CEO or housewife. We all must have daily exercise for good, healthy hearts and bodies.

Good Shoes & Socks Promote Happy Feet

Comfortable walking shoes with flexible rubber soles, particularly under the heel is important. We often insert Dr. Scholl's (our friend and follower who lived to almost 100) foam inner soles (available at shoe and drug stores). Safeguard your precious feet with good serviceable shoes and ample padding. Otherwise, the continual jarring of walking, jogging and exercising in ill-fitting or thin-soled shoes can eventually cause some foot discomfort and discouragement! Shoes should not be too loose or overly tight. Feet often swell from added stimulation and circulation caused by running and when shoes are too tight you can get painful blisters. Your socks must fit right. Make sure they haven't any holes or repairs that could cause chafing or blistering. Be sure your socks aren't the kind that bunch up inside your shoes. We often wear 2 pairs of socks – first a thin cotton pair, then a heavier wool pair – just as many tennis champs do.

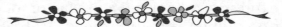

High Systolic Pressure Plays Role in Hypertension & Heart Disease

New studies from University of California, Irvine College of Medicine has found that most older patients with high blood pressure have higher than normal readings of systolic, or upper pressure, but normal lower or diastolic readings. "We were surprised to find so many patients with this pattern of blood pressure readings," stated Dr. Stanley S. Franklin, professor of medicine and lead researcher, "If more attention were paid to systolic pressure, we might see fewer people who are at a higher risk for heart disease and stroke." The researchers believe that high systolic pressure may be left untreated because most doctors assume that higher diastolic pressure indicates a greater risk of heart disease than systolic pressure. The study found that among participants aged 50 and older, about 80% had systolic blood pressure higher than 140, but had diastolic pressure below 90. (120 over 70 is ideal.)

Try and *do your jogging on grass or soft surfaces.* Grass is easier on the legs and feet, especially if you are a big person. Your legs carry you throughout life and deserve every consideration you can give them! *There might be some discomfort,* particularly if your exercise during the past years has been mostly confined to lifting a knife and fork! In addition to comfortable clothes and a good exercise space, you will need will power and a dedicated purpose to keep at it! When first starting you might be hindered by unaccustomed aches, pains and blisters. Remember, this soreness is often a healthy sign that important changes are underway in your body. Think of any temporary discomfort in this way and you'll even take pride in feeling stiff for a few days. Take a hot apple cider vinegar bath (add half cup of apple cider vinegar). The big rule to follow is, *train but don't strain.*

Alternate Running and Walking
"One step begins a ten thousand mile journey."

A wise Chinese proverb to start your new, exciting journey toward Healthy Heart Fitness with a winning attitude! One yard is approximately the longest step you can take. Now, step off 25 yards or 50, 75 or 100 and slowly increase distance and do more sets. Initially run any of these distances. If you have not been exercising, make your first weeks' daily runs 25 to 50 yards. Run or jog whatever distance you choose as a starter. After the run, then walk the same distance, briskly and breathe deeply while keeping your head and shoulders up and your arms swinging. Deep breathing is important. The reason you are doing this exercise is to give your heart more oxygen. Dad and I are faithful to our fast walking/running program. Walking/running every day helps your heart get stronger!

Wisdom is the principal thing; therefore get wisdom: and with all thy getting get understanding. – Proverbs 4:7

The medical journal Circulation *reports people who don't make efforts to exercise regularly face the same dangerous risk of heart disease as people who smoke a pack of cigarettes daily.*

Of all knowledge, that most worth having is knowledge about health. The first requisite of a good life is to be a healthy person. – Herbert Spencer

87

Daily Walk and Run Brings Miracles

When you walk and run every day, the sustained pressure on the circulatory system adds elasticity to the blood vessels, increasing their capacity for greater and easier blood flow. It's remarkable that this simple exercise can be such a positive step in protecting your heart and health. A great Heart Specialist in London told us that any person who will run 15 to 30 minutes daily for a year could expect to double the capacity of their main arteries. *This is the way to build a powerful heart.* Activity (walking, jogging, running, etc.) that causes deep breathing requires more energy. The body produces this energy by burning foodstuffs – and the burning agent is oxygen. The body can store food at each meal, using what it wants and saving some of the rest for later, but it can't store oxygen. Most of us produce enough energy to perform ordinary daily activities. But as physical activity becomes more vigorous, the unfit people just can't keep up, because the means for oxygen delivery is limited in their bodies. This is what separates the fit from the unfit!

Jogging and running demands you to breathe more oxygen in and forces your body to process and deliver it. Even if you have been inactive or sick, start simple walking and light exercise and soon it will help you to build better circulation and a more vital oxygen intake. A sound heart, like a sound car, can be driven far and fast without harm, but periods of rest and recovery are required. As we live longer, the need for rest generally increases, but not as much as most people imagine. A daily 20 to 30 minute nap is an ideal recharger after lunch.

> **Like a car, regular maintenance and sensible use can keep the heart working in an *as new* condition even at a vintage age.**

To maintain good health the body must be exercised properly (walking, jogging, running, biking, swimming, deep breathing, good posture, etc.) and nourished wisely (natural foods), so as to provide and increase the good life of radiant health, joy, peace and happiness. – Paul C. Bragg

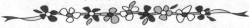

There is no thrill quite like doing something you didn't know you could.
– Marjorie Holmes

Chapter 10

Exercise For Health and Good Circulation

Good Circulation – Key to Strong Heart

When any part of the circulatory system is seriously impaired, the billions of body cells it serves are deprived of their oxygen and nourishment. With their blood supply cut off, these cells will automatically break down. The cell damage may occur in the heart itself and in the brain, the lungs, kidneys, skin or other parts of the body. Remember – if you don't use your body, you will lose it!

Five Exercises for Increased Circulation

Exercise 1 – Windmill Exercise For Energy

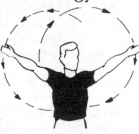

(A) Stand erect with heels and toes together, chest up, stomach drawn in, shoulders back, head high, with hands hanging loosely at your sides. Now, start swinging your arms in a forward circular motion then coming down along the sides of your body, continuing circles. Increase speed until you are making circles as fast as possible. Start by doing 10 circles forward and increase by several a day until you can bring it up to 30 circles at one time.

(B) Same position as above, only instead of making circles with the arms forward, make circles backward – in the opposite direction. Start with 10 and increase to 30.

Exercise 2 – Hands and Finger Circulation Exercise

Stand erect as in Exercise #1. Bring hands 10 inches in front of body at chest height, and from the wrists shake the relaxed hands vigorously. Do 15 shakes with both hands at the same time and then grip hands together 15 times. Now 15 times grip each hand individually into a tight fist, then relax the hands, stretching fingers out as far as possible.

Each day is God's gift to you. Make it blossom and grow into a thing of beauty.

89

Exercise 3 – Body Circulation-Builder

This exercise is great for people in cold climates to bring circulation to their arms, hands and upper body. Start in the same position as Exercise #1. Hold arms and hands outstretched horizontally at shoulder height. Each hand forms a half circle as the exercise is done. The right hand strikes the left shoulder and the left hand strikes the right shoulder at the same time. The arms are crisscrossed alternately with each repetition . . . right over left and then left over right. Slap the shoulders vigorously. Make it vigorous so each time the arms are flung open back to the starting position, then the chest is pushed forward and up. Start this exercise by doing it 10 times and work up until you can do it 30 times.

Exercise 4 – Leg and Feet Vibrating Exercise

Stand erect, feet about 8 to 10 inches apart and arms at sides. Now, put all your weight on your left foot and raise your right foot off the ground about 6 or 8 inches. Make short stretching kicks in a forward direction. (You may hold on to a chair.) You will feel vibration from the hips to the toes. Now alternate, standing on right foot and kicking with your left foot. Start with 10 kicks on each foot and increase the amount every day until you can kick about 30 times or more with each foot. Make this a vigorous exercise – it promotes great circulation to hips, thighs, calves and feet and is important for health.

Exercise 5 – Exercise for Blood Circulation in Head

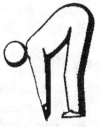

Stand erect with knees relaxed and feet 12 inches apart. Lean forward from waist, with arms hanging down, relaxed near floor. (Hold on to chair if necessary.) In this position gently roll your head side to side and down and up. Do this exercise only a few times in the beginning, until your neck and head becomes accustomed to more circulation.

These simple exercises cause no heart strain and are ideal for improving circulation. They help open up blocked arteries and blood vessels. When circulation is increased through exercise it helps purify the blood so more oxygen is carried to all parts of the body.

Exercises – Good For Heart and Health

A normal, healthy heart cannot be injured by these exercises. Weak people should start slowly and work up to a vigorous workout. Just as exercise is good for any muscle, these circulatory exercises are beneficial for both a healthy and an injured heart. These exercises will condition your heart just as they do your visible muscles. Refuse to listen to people who try to frighten you away from exercise! The heart is a muscle and must be exercised if it is to remain strong. By exercising you will build a stronger heart and body!

Do these exercises daily – requires only 15 minutes. This is just a little time to invest in a healthy heart and a healthful life! If you have a sedentary job, if you spend a lot of time sitting or standing, do these exercises 2 or 3 times daily. When on long automobile drives, stop and do exercises every few hours. The more you do these exercises, the better circulation you will have, and this promotes a stronger heart! When at home, after your exercises you can enjoy the Special Shower as below.

Special Shower Builds Healthy Circulation

Here's a progressive method for improving circulation over your entire body. All you need is a large back brush or Swedish bath friction mitt, castile soap and a coarse Turkish towel. Get into shower and turn on the hot water. With brush or mitt, gently scrub your body. At first your coddled body won't be able to take too much scrubbing. Also it's good to hand–massage neck and upper shoulders. After your scrub/massage part, then alternate hot or cold showers (*filtered) for 3 to 5 minutes. Now towel rub dry your body for 3 to 5 minutes – your circulation will tingle!

It's wonderful relaxation for tired or sore muscles and refreshing stimulation with the hot/cold water shower, letting the spray beat heavily on back and shoulders. Occasionally before shower apply olive oil if skin is dry. We advise this relaxing shower before dinner on days when you come home tired. It refreshes and relaxes you!

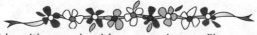

*Don't gamble with your health, use a shower filter to remove toxins. To get info on the best shower filter available call 800-446-1990. I have been using this filter for 3 years and enjoy my safe, chlorine-free showers!

Exercise to Benefit the Liver and Kidneys

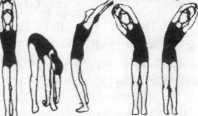

Your great filters – the kidneys – are the body's hardest working organs! Exercises that bend and twist the body at its middle will help to stimulate the kidneys, which makes them function more efficiently.

Here's a great exercise for stimulating the kidneys:

Stand up straight with hands over head. Now bend forward from waist with knees relaxed and try to touch toes. Return your hands overhead, now bend backwards as far as comfortable. Now, arms up, hands clasped, bend first to left side, then to right side as far as possible. Since most of the body's liquid waste is eliminated through the kidneys, you should do these kidney stimulating exercises daily. Start with 10 of each and work up to 30.

The Dangers of Sitting too Long

Although most waste products are eliminated through the kidneys, the lungs expel carbon dioxide. In the tiny alveoli of the lungs, blood discharges carbon dioxide and takes on oxygen, again turning a bright red. It then flows back into the heart, to be pumped out through the arteries to the rest of the body. This powerful cycle is repeated thousands of times each day. This is the reason you must never sit too long at one time. *Sitting slows down the circulation and stagnates the blood.* Long periods of sitting can be damaging to the heart. And please, never cross your legs – it's unhealthy!

People who sit too long may develop a thrombosis (blood clot) in the deep veins of the calf. If your office work requires sitting a lot, *get up and move around every hour.* On long car trips, stop every hour or so and take a walk or do some exercises. Remember when exercising, you flush out toxins and stimulate blood circulation through your vital pipes that supply food and oxygen.

Cheerfulness is the atmosphere under which all things thrive. – Jean Paul Richter

The Art of Healthy Sitting

When sitting, sit correctly! *The most disastrous and injurious habit of bad sitting is crossing the legs* for it compresses the popliteal artery in the back of the knees which can cause a variety of unhealthy problems (blood stagnation – leg, hip and backaches, varicose veins, hemorrhoids, headaches, pain, etc.).

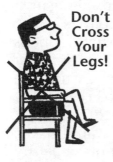
Don't Cross Your Legs!

When you sit in a chair, sit well back. Do not let the edge of the chair cut off circulation in the back of the knees. Keep your feet on floor. Dangling your legs puts too much pressure on veins. When I was small, my dad shortened the legs of a table for me so that my feet would touch the floor. Adults who have shorter legs should use a footstool. We love rocking chairs – you can get rest by sitting, plus some peaceful (even problem solving) rocking exercise!

Sweating is Healthy for You!

The skin, with its millions of pores and sweat glands, is the body's largest eliminating organ – (often called the third kidney). Sweat has a dual purpose – it rids the body of impurities and serves as a temperature regulator. When our body is exposed to heat or *warmed up* by exercise, sweat glands are stimulated into action. Evaporation of the sweat cools the blood when it reaches the skin. This helps the body from becoming overheated and, at the same time, eliminates impurities near the skin's surface.

It's the toxic impurities or the mixture with skin dirt, that gives sweat a bad odor. If you are clean inside and out, then there is only the good sweat smell. Regardless of what deodorant advertisers say, *it's healthy to sweat.* From dancing, calisthenics, walking, cycling and even vigorous housework, to saunas and steam rooms – any activity that makes you sweat improves your heart action and health. Hard work never hurts when you're healthy!

Nervous Tension can ruin your health in dozens of ways, diminish your productivity and even shorten your lifespan. – Dr. E. Jacobson, You Must Relax

Indulge in Hobbies That Are Active and Fun

My dad said if he were the President of the United States he would advocate laws requiring all people who work sitting down to spend an equal amount of time in keeping physically fit by brisk walking, etc. Also TV or computer addicts would be required to spend an hour in brisk walking for every hour they sit before a screen.

We would like to start a healthy-heart crusade against inactivity, long sitting and sedentary activities. Long sitting slows down circulation and when that happens many changes take place in the artery walls. You must keep active! When you relax, relax actively. Cultivate hobbies that give you needed exercise that you can enjoy such as hiking, swimming, tennis, golf, etc. You can't build a strong heart unless you exercise, walk briskly, bend, twist, vibrate your body, which promotes healthy overall body circulation. Stagnation breeds disease.

Avoid Constricting Clothes and Shoes

Anything that impedes blood circulation damages the heart and its arterial and vascular systems. Therefore, wear no constricting under garments – this includes *tight bras, belts, collars, ties and above all, tight shoes.

Tight shoes can do more to disturb the circulation than any other article of clothing because the feet must always be well supplied with blood. There are 26 bones in each foot – more than in any other part of the body. When the blood does not reach the feet in the required quantities, toxins are retained in the cell structures of the feet. That is why so many people's feet have an unpleasant odor – they need to detoxify their body.

Many conditions of stiffness and deformities are brought on by ill-fitting shoes that cause poor circulation and incorrect posture when walking and standing. Only wear comfortable, practical shoes that don't bind or inhibit the free circulation of the blood to the feet.

* Read *Dressed to Kill*, by Sydney Singer, on breast cancer and bra studies. Call (800) 788-6262 to order this revealing book.

Slow down and enjoy life. It's not only the scenery you miss by going too fast – you also miss the sense of where you're going and why. – Eddie Cantor

Exercise Helps Build Better Circulation To Your Feet, Hands and Whole Body

Walking barefoot is the ideal way to walk. Each time we remove our shoes and walk barefoot is an opportunity to improve our circulation and walk toward more fitness for our heart. Walking on the grass, walking on the sand, earth or simply walking barefoot around the house improves circulation and helps strengthen the heart.

The heart must pump blood to the legs and feet, as well as to the arms and hands. Most people do not have sufficient rhythmic circulation to these extremities. That is why so many people complain of cold or numb feet, legs that *go to sleep* easily and arms and hands that become cold and numb. Here is a hydrotherapeutic water method that alleviates these conditions:

Cold and Hot Water Circulation Therapy:

Get 2 small foot tubs or wash tubs. Fill one with hot water – about 104° or as hot as you can stand. Fill the other with cold water, preferably with ice cubes added. Now for 2 minutes put your feet in the hot water and your entire lower arms (hands to elbows) submerged in the cold water. After 2 minutes reverse the procedure – put your feet in the cold water, your arms and hands in the hot water for another 2 minute period. Repeat this cycle 5 times, then take a coarse cotton towel and rub your feet, arms and hands vigorously until they are warm and glowing with tingling, healthy circulation.

95

Here's another super therapy to stimulate circulation in the feet. Sit on a chair next to a bathtub with feet dangling over the tub; turn on a strong flow of water and for 5 minutes, alternate hot and cold water over your feet. Finish up with coarse towel rub and massage.

Exercise Gives Huge Benefits for the Prevention of Heart Disease and also:

1. Tones muscles
2. Improves circulation
3. Lowers cholesterol
4. Chases Depression
5. Eases stress
6. Stimulates internal organs
7. Improves sex
8. Promotes sound sleep
9. Helps you think better
10. Promotes deep breathing

Great Framingham 50 Year Heart Study

In 1948 in Framingham, Massachusetts, 2,336 men and 2,873 women were recruited into a landmark study, the Framingham Heart Study. This ongoing study is still the source of much of our present understanding of heart disease and stroke. The original study group of 1948 and the succeeding generation of Framingham residents have been followed throughout their lives. Everyone has been interviewed and examined every 2 years for over 50 years. This massive pioneer medical research continues today.

In 1971, the original Framingham subjects were joined by 5,135 of their children. The researchers were pleased to find a 43% reduction in coronary heart disease death from the 1948 group. Our favorite – *The New England Journal of Medicine* says the increasing heart-health of Framingham's 1970s test group is primarily the result of the lifestyle improvements (cholesterol, blood pressure and smoking factors) that so harmed the early 1950s group. See website: *http://mayohealth.org/mayo/9902/htm/framingh.htm*

Dr. T. Colin Campbell's China Project

In another landmark study, the China Project, written by Dr. T. Colin Campbell, the effects of nearly 50 disease categories on rural and urban counties (in US and China) were observed for 20 years. Results showed that populations using a diet richer in animal products and higher in total fat were much more afflicted with chronic degenerative diseases (cancers, cardiovascular diseases, diabetes, etc.). The Chinese diet contains from 0 to 20% animal-based foods, while the affluent American diet, *sad to say*, is comprised of 50 to 70%. What's worse, far more Americans are clinically obese, even though the Chinese consume 30% more total calories! Another astonishing fact is that China's high cholesterol levels are almost equal to the U.S.'s low! See *www.newcenturynutrition. com/china_project/index.html* for more info on this study!

What these 2 ambitious studies have to say about maintaining cardiovascular health is just what we've been telling you for years! Eat a natural diet low in cholesterol, fats, sugars and salts, etc.; exercise regularly, fast and don't smoke – this is The Bragg Healthy Lifestyle!

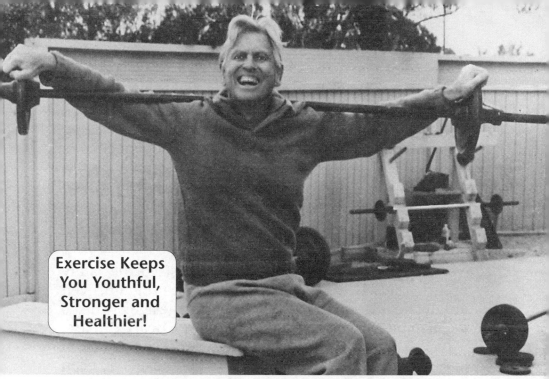

Paul C. Bragg and Patricia lift weights 3 times weekly.

Iron-Pumping Oldsters (ages 86 to 96) Triple Their Muscle Strength In Landmark U.S. Government Study

WASHINGTON, June 13, 1990 — Ageing nursing home residents in Boston *pumping iron?* Elderly weightlifters tripling and quadrupling their muscle strength? Is it possible? Most people would doubt and wonder at this amazing revelation!

Yet government experts on ageing answered those questions with a resounding *yes* according to results of a new study. They turned a group of frail Boston nursing home residents, aged 86 to 96, into weightlifters to demonstrate that it's never too late to reverse age-related declines in muscle strength. The study group participated in a regime of high-intensity weight-training in research conducted by the Agriculture Departments Human 1 Research Center of Ageing at Tufts University in Boston. *A high-intensity weight training program is capable of inducing dramatic increases in muscle strength in frail men and women up to 96 years of age,* reported Dr. Maria A. Fiatarone, who was the Study Director.

Amazing Health & Fitness Results in 8 Weeks

The favorable response to strength training in these subjects was remarkable in light of their very advanced age, extremely sedentary habits, many chronic diseases, functional disabilities and nutritional inadequacies.

Despite their many handicaps, the elderly weight lifters increased their muscle strength by 3 to 4 times as much in as little as 8 weeks. Fiatarone said they probably were stronger at the end of the program than they had been in years! *www.cchs.usyd.edu.au/ESS/fiatarone/research.html*

Fiatarone and her associates emphasized the safety of such a closely supervised weight lifting program, even among people in frail health. The average age of the 10 participants was 90. Six had coronary heart disease, 7 had arthritis, 6 had bone fractures resulting from osteoporosis, 4 had high blood pressure, and all had been physically inactive for years. Yet no serious medical problems resulted from this program. A few of the participants did report minor muscle and joint aches, but 9 of the 10 still completed the program. One man, aged 86, felt a pulling sensation at the site of a previous hernia incision and dropped out after 4 weeks.

The study participants, drawn from a 712 bed long-term care facility in Boston, worked out 3 times a week during the study. They performed 3 sets of 8 repetitions with each leg on a weight lifting machine. The weights were gradually increased from 10 pounds to about 40 pounds at the end of the 8 week program.

Fiatarone said the study carries potentially important implications for older people, who represent a growing proportion of the population. A decline in muscle strength and size is one of the more predictable features of ageing. Muscle strength in the average adult decreases by 30% to 50% during the course of a lifetime. Experts on ageing do not know whether the decrease is an unavoidable consequence of ageing, or results mainly from sedentary lifestyle and other controllable factors.

Exercise, along with some fasting helps maintain or restore a healthy physical balance and normal weight for a long, happy life.

Muscle atrophy and weakness is not merely a cosmetic problem in elderly people, especially the frail elderly. Researchers have linked muscle weakness with recurrent falls, which is a major cause of immobility and death with the American elderly. This is costing the United States billions of dollars yearly in staggering medical fees.

Previous studies have suggested that weight training can be helpful in reversing age-related muscle weakness. But Fiatarone said physicians have been reluctant to recommend weight lifting for frail elderly patients with multiple health problems. This new government study might help to change their minds. Also, this study shows the great importance of keeping the 640 body muscles as active and fit as possible to maintain general good physical fitness and also good heart and body health.

20 Year Study Shows Being Fit Saves Money

The average American spends over $4,000 on health care yearly, and costs are rising: Private health-insurance premiums jumped 8.2% in 1998, more than twice as much as in the previous years (3.3% in 1996, 3.5% in 1997). This revealing 20 year study done by Dr. Ted Mitchell of The Cooper Clinic in Texas monitored 6,679 men. Results showed those who exercised more, required fewer doctor visits. Being fit cuts yearly medical expenses 25 to 60%. Study also found all you need to stay fit is to exercise just 20 to 30 minutes a day, four or five days a week. Physically fit people live longer and enjoy a better quality of life! www.cooperaerobics.com

99

Excerpt from Bragg *Miracle of Fasting*:

Dr. Nikolayev, Director of a famous European fasting clinic, often quotes an old German proverb:

"The illness that can't be cured by fasting can't be cured by anything else."
Fasting permits the miracle cleansing and healing powers of the body and of the mind to assert themselves.

Dr. Nikolayev – who fasts several times a year in 7, 10 to 15 day stretches stated, "I usually fast for prophylactic reasons. I have fasted several times with a scientific purpose in view, to make an experiment. I always feel excellent when I fast. It is always a happy, restful occasion."

Dr. Nikolayev discovered that his patients responded to fasting treatment after all other forms of therapy had failed. The patients had been chronically ill and felt hopeless about their future! Most of them would never have functioned again. Fasting gave them a new fresh lease on life.

Allan Cott, M.D. noted in his book – *Fasting, The Ultimate Diet* that "75% of patients treated by fasting improved so remarkably that they were able to resume an active life!" See our Dr. Fasting chapter on pages 155-161.

KEEP BIOLOGICALLY HEALTHY & YOUTHFUL WITH EXERCISE & GOOD NUTRITION

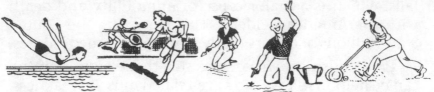

Always remember you have the following important reasons for following The Bragg Healthy Lifestyle:

- The ironclad laws of Mother Nature and God.
- Your common sense, which tells you that you are doing right.
- Your aim to make your health better and your life longer.
- Your resolve to prevent illness so that you may enjoy life.
- Make an art of healthy living; you will be youthful at any age.
- You will retain your faculties and be hale, hearty, active and useful far beyond the ordinary length of years.
- You will also possess superior mental and physical powers!

100

WANTED – For Robbing Health & Life

KILLER Saturated Fats   CHOKER Hydrogenated Fats
CLOGGER Salt   DEADEYED Devitalized Foods
DOPEY Caffeine   HARD WATER Inorganic Minerals
PLUGGER Frying Pan   JERKY Turbulent Emotions
DEATH-DEALER Drugs   CRAZY Alcohol
GREASY Obesity   SMOKY Tobacco
HOGGY Overeating   LOAFER Laziness

What Wise Men Say

Wisdom does not show itself so much in precept as in life – a firmness of mind and mastery of appetite. – Seneca

I saw few die of hunger – of eating, a hundred thousand. – Ben Franklin

Govern well thy appetite, lest Sin surprise thee, & her black attendant, Death. – Milton

Thy food shall be thy remedy. – Hippocrates

Our prayers should be for a sound mind in a healthy body. – Juvenal

Health is…a blessing that money cannot buy. – Izaak Walton

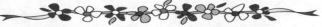

The natural healing force within us is the greatest force in getting well. – Hippocrates, Father of Medicine

Of all the knowledge, that most worth having is the knowledge about health! The first requisite of a good life is to be a healthy person. – Herbert Spencer

Chapter 11

Doctor Pure Water

Pure Water Helps Keep Body Clean Inside

To have a clean, healthy bloodstream and arteries free from encrustation and corrosion, we must not only eat correctly but also drink the right fluids. *The liquids which go into our bodies must be pure and nourishing.*

To begin with, we believe that every person should have the equivalent of *8 to 10 glasses of pure distilled water every day.* It can be obtained in most supermarkets, grocery stores and health stores. If you cannot find it readily, look under *water* in the yellow pages of your telephone directory for local bottled water suppliers.

Distilled water has no inorganic minerals to deposit on the walls of the arteries and other *pipes* of the body. In contrast, most sources of *well, spring and river waters all contain inorganic minerals and some even have toxic chemicals which cannot ever be utilized in the body chemistry.* They corrode the human *pipes* just as they do the plumbing pipes which bring water into your home.

101

Hard Water Causes Hard Arteries

The human body has a vast piping system called the bloodstream. A healthy heart must have clean, open coronary arteries. The blood must be able to flow through them smoothly to nourish the heart and keep it pumping steadily and efficiently.

Suppose a person drinks only the hard chemicalized water (as most people do) and their pipelines become clogged and blocked by the inorganic minerals which can't be absorbed into the body. Blockage in the coronary arteries that feed the heart reduces the amount of blood reaching the heart. When the blood supply is reduced enough, the affected parts of the heart cease to function. *Heart attacks and even death may result when some sections of the heart muscle stop functioning.*

Pure water is the best drink for a wise man. – Henry David Thoreau

Your Arteries Are Your Lifeline

Blockages can be life-threatening. They have serious health consequences that can occur not only in the heart's arteries, but throughout the entire arterial system. If blockage occurs in the arteries going to the brain, a stroke occurs and paralysis and even death may result.

Arteriosclerosis, or hardening of the arteries, means that the arteries have become brittle and lost their elasticity due to injurious deposits in the artery walls. The entire pipe system may become so blocked that the blood carrying oxygen and nourishment to the cells of the body and its vital organs, cannot get through, or flow that does manage to squeeze through is insufficient.

Most people want to blame hardening of the arteries on their calendar years. But calendar years don't put those inorganic minerals into the arteries. *Time is not toxic* and time is not a force that damages the body. Time is a measurement and nothing else. *Don't blame your years for your physical troubles!* You can only blame yourself for not taking care of your miracle body that God has given you. (It's seldom ever too late to change and improve.)

The Difference Between Organic and Inorganic Minerals

Inorganic minerals never lived and are inert . . . which means that they *cannot be absorbed into the body!*

Organic minerals are those which come from that which is *living* or has lived . . . and *16 of these organic minerals are essential elements of the human body.* When we eat an apple or any other fruit or vegetable, that substance is living, for it has a certain lifespan after it has been picked. The same is true of animal foods, such as fish, milk, cheese and eggs. Animals obtain their organic minerals from plants. We humans obtain our organic minerals from both plants and animals.

Angina, allergies, asthma, back and joint pains, migraines, stomach pains and arthritis may all be symptoms of severe dehydration – which can easily be helped by drinking 8 to 10 glasses of pure distilled water daily! Start increasing your water intake today. Be water wise and health safe! – Paul C. Bragg

Only a living plant has the power to extract inorganic minerals from the earth and sun and change them into organic minerals. No animal or human can do this. If you were stranded on an uninhabited island where nothing was growing, you would starve to death. Although the soil beneath your feet would contain all 16 *essential* minerals, your body could not absorb them.

Organic minerals are vital in keeping us alive and healthy, but inorganic minerals can stiffen, sicken and slowly kill us!

Many years ago my father was on an expedition in China when one part of the country was suffering from drought and famine. He saw the poor, starving people heating and eating dirt for want of food. They died horrible deaths because they could not get one bit of nourishment from the inorganic minerals of the earth.

Hard Water is Unhealthy

For years we've heard people claim that certain waters were rich in all the minerals. What minerals are they talking about? Inorganic or organic? If they are inorganic, people are simply burdening their bodies with inert minerals which may cause the development of stones in the kidneys and gall bladder and acid crystals in the arteries, veins, joints and other parts of the body.

Dad was reared in a part of Virginia known for its extremely *hard water.* The drinking water was heavily saturated with inorganic minerals – especially sodium, iron and calcium. He saw many of his adult relations and friends die of kidney trouble. Nearly all the people were prematurely old because the inorganic minerals had collected on the inner walls of their arteries and veins. These people would often die from hardening of the arteries. One of Dad's uncles died at the great Johns Hopkins Hospital in Baltimore, Maryland, when he was only 48 years of age. The doctors who performed the autopsy stated that his arteries were so corroded with inorganic minerals that they were as hard as clay pipes!

Most Americans' bodies thirst for pure distilled water! Their bodies become sick, prematurely aged, crippled and stiff due to inorganic minerals and chemicalized water and lack of sufficient pure water!

Vegetable and Fruit Juices Contain Mother Nature's Distilled Water

No new water has been put on the face of Mother Earth since it was originally formed. Just as the same energy is formed and re-formed, so the same water is used and re-used over and over again by the miracle of Mother Nature. Waters of the earth are purified by distillation. The sun evaporates the water which is collected into clouds. When the clouds become full we have rain and dew – pure, perfectly clean, distilled water, free of all harmful inorganic substances, until polluted!

Years ago, when the late Douglas Fairbanks, Senior, and Dad were close friends, they roamed the South Sea Islands for several months. During that trip Dad came upon an island inhabited by *beautiful, healthy Polynesians* who drank only distilled water because the island was surrounded by the Pacific Ocean. Their island was based on porous coral which could not hold water – so they would *only drink rain water* or the fresh, clear, clean water of the green coconut. Dad had never seen any finer specimens of humanity than these native South Sea Islanders. There were several doctors on the yacht who thoroughly examined the most mature people on these islands. One heart doctor stated that he had never in his life examined such healthy, well-preserved people.

You may have noted we said only the most mature people were examined by the doctors. *They were so completely unaware of age* that no such word existed in their language! They never celebrated birthdays, so they were forever young – gloriously ageless, not only in years but in body. These older men performed as well in the vigorous native dances as the younger men. They were all beautiful human specimens because they lived their lengthy lives drinking only pure distilled water, eating natural foods and enjoying a healthy lifestyle.

The great thing in life is not so much where you stand, but in what direction you are moving.

Former U.S. Surgeon General Koop warned Americans in a landmark 1988 report on Nutrition and Health that diet-related diseases account for 68% of deaths!

Why We Drink Only Distilled Water

Sadly, in some areas it's no longer safe to drink rain or snow water because of man's vast reach of polluting the air. But when you drink the fresh juices of fruits and vegetables, remember that all of this liquid has been *distilled by Mother Nature* and is 100% inorganic mineral-free. Fresh fruit and vegetable juices contain Mother Nature's pure distilled water, plus important nutrients such as natural sugars, organic minerals and vitamins.

You will hear people say, *distilled water is dead water, a fish cannot live in it.* Of course a fish cannot live in distilled water for any length of time! It needs the vegetation that grows in rivers, lakes and seas. But this doesn't mean it isn't the very best of all waters to drink.

Another erroneous notion about distilled water is that it *leaches the organic minerals out of the body.* This is 100% false. It leaches out the inorganic minerals which you want to be rid of that cause painful health problems.

Distilled water helps to dissolve and flush out the terrible toxic poisons that collect in the bodies of modern man. This pure water helps to eliminate these toxic poisons through the kidneys without creating painful problems that inorganic pebbles and stones do!

Every liquid prescription that is mixed in any drug store the world over is prepared with distilled water. It is used in baby formulas and for many hundreds of other purposes where absolutely pure water is essential.

Distilled water is soft water. If you wash your hair in distilled water you will discover how soft it is.

There are water softeners being used in millions of homes because hard water is not ideal for washing clothes, dishes, etc. Please do not drink the water that comes out of water softeners! It's not healthy water for drinking or cooking because of its salt and chemical content.

At the Bragg home we have a water distiller and for our office staff we have distilled water delivered in 5 gallon bottles. Try distilled water exclusively for a year, you will see the results and never drink hard water again!

WATER IS KEY TO HEALTH & ALL BODY FUNCITONS

- Heart
- Circulation
- Digestion
- Bones & Joints
- Muscles
- Metabolism
- Assimilation
- Elimination
- Nerves
- Energy
- Sex
- Glands

The body is 70% water and pure, steam-distilled (chemical-free) water is important for total health. You should drink at least 8 glasses of water daily. Read our book, Water – The Shocking Truth, for more info on the importance of pure water. See back pages for book list.

Pure, distilled water is vitally important in following The Bragg Healthy Lifestyle. Water is the key to all body functions including: digestion, circulation, bones and joints, assimilation, elimination, muscles, nerves, glands, sex and senses. The right kind of water is one of your best natural protections against all kinds of diseases and viral infections, such as influenza and pneumonia. It is a vital factor in all body fluids, tissues, cells, lymph, blood and all glandular secretions. Water holds all nutritive factors in solution, as well as toxins and body wastes, and acts as the main transportation medium throughout the body, for both nutritional and cleansing purposes!

106

Distilled water is the world's purest and best water!

It's excellent for detoxification, fasting and cleansing of the cells, organs and fluids of the body because it helps carry away the harmful toxins, substances, etc.

Water from chemically treated public water systems – and even from many wells and springs – is likely to be loaded with poisonous chemicals and toxic trace elements. Depending upon the kinds of pipes used in the buildings, the water is likely to be overloaded with lead (from older, soldered pipe joints), zinc (from old-fashioned galvanized pipes) or with copper and cadmium (from copper pipes). These trace elements are released in dangerous quantities by the chemical action of the water flowing against the metals of the pipes.

Distilled water plays vital part in treatment of illness, arthritis, etc. – Dr. Banik

There is only one water that is clean and that is steam distilled water. No other substance on our planet does so much to keep us healthy and get us well as this water does. – Dr. James Balch, *Dietary Wellness*

The 70% Watery Human

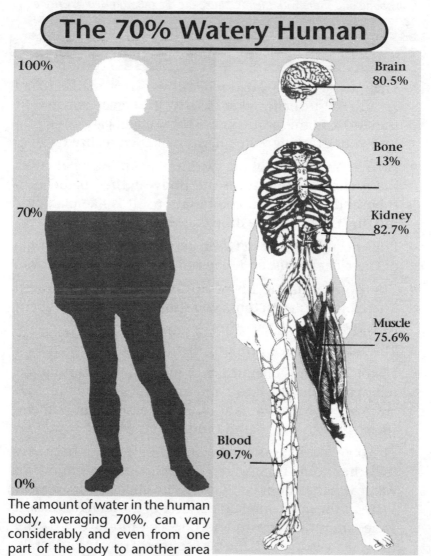

100%

70%

0%

Brain
80.5%

Bone
13%

Kidney
82.7%

Muscle
75.6%

Blood
90.7%

The amount of water in the human body, averaging 70%, can vary considerably and even from one part of the body to another area (illustration on right). A lean man may hold 70% of his weight in body water, while a woman – because of her larger proportion of water-poor fatty tissues – may be only 52% water. The lowering of the water content in the blood is what triggers the hypothalamus, the brain's thirst center, to send out its familiar urgent demand for a drink of water.

Water Percentage in Various Body Parts:

Teeth	10%	Lungs	80%
Bones	13%	Brain	80.5%
Cartilage	55%	Bile	86%
Red blood corpuscles	68.7%	Plasma	90%
Liver	71.5%	Blood	90.7%
Muscle tissue	75%	Lymph	94%
Spleen	75.5%	Saliva	95.5%

Pure water is the essential fluid of life.

Ten Common Sense Reasons Why You Should Only Drink Pure, Distilled Water!

- There are over 12,000 toxic chemicals on the market today . . . and 500 are being added yearly! Wherever you live, in the city or on the farm, some of these chemicals are getting into your drinking water. Beware of chemicalized water.

- No one on the face of the earth today knows what effect these chemicals have on the body as they blend into thousands of different combinations. It is like making a mixture of colors; one drop could change the color.

- Proper equipment hasn't been designed yet to detect some of these chemicals, and may not be for years to come.

- The body is made up of approximately 70% water. Therefore, don't you think you should be particular about the type of water you drink?

- The Navy has been drinking distilled water for years!

- Distilled water is chemical and mineral free. Distillation removes all the chemicals and impurities from water that are possible to remove. If distillation doesn't remove them, there is no known method today that will.

- The body does need minerals . . . but it is not necessary that they come from water. There is not one mineral in water which cannot be found more abundantly in food! Water is the most unreliable source of minerals because it varies from one area to another. The food we eat – not the water we drink – is the best source of organic minerals!

- Distilled water is used for intravenous feeding, inhalation therapy, prescriptions and baby formulas. Therefore, doesn't it make sense that it is good for everyone?

- Thousands of water distillers have been sold throughout the United States and around the world to individuals, families, dentists, doctors, hospitals, nursing homes and government agencies. These informed, alert consumers are helping protect their health by using only steam distilled water. They don't want toxic chemicals.

- With chemicals, pollutants and other impurities in our water, it makes good sense to clean up the water you drink using Mother Nature's inexpensive way – distillation.

Fluorine is a Deadly Poison!

Millions of innocent people have been brainwashed by the aluminum companies to erroneously believe that adding sodium fluoride (their waste by-product) to our drinking water will reduce tooth decay in our children. Americans get sodium fluoride in their drinking water without thinking about it. Sodium fluorine, a chemical "cousin" of sodium fluoride, is used as a rat and roach killer and a deadly pesticide. Yet this deadly sodium fluoride, injected almost by government edict into drinking water in the proportion of 1.2 parts per million (PPM), has been declared by the US Public Health Service to be *safe for all human consumption.* Every chemist knows that such *absolute safety* is not only false and is truly unattainable, but a total illusion!

Keep Toxic Fluoride Out of Your Water!

Most of the water Americans drink has fluoride in it, including tap, bottled and canned drinks and foods! The ADA (American Dental Association) is insisting that the FDA (Food and Drug Association) mandate the addition of fluoride to all bottled waters! Defend your right to drink pure, nonfluoridated tap and bottled waters! Challenge and stop local and state water fluoridation policies! Call, write, fax or e-mail all your state officials and Congress people and send them a copy of this book.

CHECK FOLLOWING WEBSITES FOR FLUORIDE UPDATES:

- www.fluoride-journal.com • www.bragg.com
- www.webaxs.net/~noel/fluoride.htm • www.saveteeth.org
- www.fluoridation.com • www.tldp.com/fluoride.htm
- emporium.turnpike.net/P/PDHA/health.htm
- www.bruha.com/fluoride/html/fluoride_and_fluoridation.htm
- www.gjne.com/cfsdwh • www.inter-view.net/~sherrell

These Eleven Major American Associations
Stopped Endorsing Water Fluoridation back in 1996

- *American Heart Assoc.* • *American Academy of Allergy & Immunology*
- *American Cancer Society* • *Chronic Fatigue Syndrome Action Network*
- *American Diabetes Assoc.* • *National Institute of Law Municipal Officers*
- *American Chiropractic Assoc.* • *American Civil Liberties Union* • *Soc. of Toxicology*
- *National Kidney Foundation* • *American Psychiatric Association*

Showers, Toxic Chemicals & Chlorine

Skin absorption of toxic contaminants has been underestimated and ingestion may not constitute the sole or even primary route of exposure.
– Dr. Halina Brown, *American Journal of Public Health*

Taking long hot showers is a health risk, according to the latest research. Showers – and to a lesser extent baths – lead to a greater exposure to toxic chemicals contained in water supplies than does drinking the water. These toxic chemicals evaporate out of the water and are inhaled. They can also spread through the house and be inhaled by others. People get six to 100 times more chemicals by breathing the air around showers and baths than they would by drinking the water.
– Ian Anderson, *New Scientist*

A professor of Water Chemistry at the University of Pittsburgh claims that exposure to vaporized chemicals in the water through showering, bathing and inhalation is 100 times greater than through drinking the water.
– *The Nader Report – Troubled Waters on Tap*

Chlorine is the greatest crippler and killer of modern times. While it prevented epidemics of one disease, it was creating another. Twenty years after the start of chlorinating our drinking water in 1904, the present epidemic of heart trouble, cancer and senility began.
– Dr. Joseph Price, *Coronaries/Cholesterol/Chlorine*

Keep World's Plant Seeds Alive – Not Sterile!
Terminator Sterile Seeds Threaten Food Freedom!

Terminator seeds are sterile crop seeds patented and marketed by the Monsanto Corp. that have been biologically altered to sprout a permanently infertile plant. The large scale use of these seeds (which is already underway in over 78 countries) could directly threaten the well-being of 1.4 billion people who now depend on food grown with fertile seeds. This would present a huge risk to the world because it could spread and sterilize all living plants, trees, etc. Farmers (and their neighbors, with plants 'accidently' cross-pollinated by Terminator plants) would be forced to buy new seeds every year. For many of these farmers financial ruin would result and bring on misery and famine for millions worldwide. Monsanto's seed program has no benefits for the world – only for the company's pocketbook. Discover Monsanto's fiendish plot to control the world's seed industry. Websites: rafi.org and sedos.org/Food/terminator.html

Five Hidden Toxic Dangers in Your Shower:

● **Chlorine:** Added to all municipal water supplies, this disinfectant hardens arteries, destroys proteins in the body, irritates skin and sinus conditions and aggravates any asthma, allergies and respiratory problems.

● **Chloroform:** This powerful by-product of chlorination causes excessive free radical formation (a cause of accelerated ageing!), normal cells to mutate and cholesterol to form. It's a known carcinogen!

● **DCA (Dichloroacedic acid):** This chlorine by-product alters cholesterol metabolism and has been shown to cause liver cancer in lab animals.

● **MX (toxic chlorinated acid):** Another by-product of chlorination, MX is known to cause genetic mutations that can lead to cancer growth and has been found in all chlorinated water for which it was tested.

● **Proven cause of bladder and rectal cancer:** Research proved that chlorinated water is the direct cause of 9% of all U.S. bladder cancers and 15% of all rectal cancers.

111

Don't Gamble With Your Health – Use Shower Filter That Removes Toxins

The most effective method of removing hazards from your shower is the quick and easy installation of a filter on your shower arm. The best filter we found removes chlorine, lead, mercury, iron, chlorine by-products, arsenic, hydrogen sulfide, and many other unseen toxic contaminants, such as bacteria, fungi, dirt and sediments. It has a 12 to 18 month filter life-span and the filter is easily cleaned by backwashing and replaced when needed. I have been using this filter for 3 years and really enjoy my chlorine-free showers! For info on buying the best shower filter call (800) 446-1990 weekdays.

Start enjoying safe, chlorine-free showers right away. It's essential to reducing your risk of heart disease and cancer and to ease the strain on your immune system. And you may even get rid of long-standing conditions – from sinus and respiratory problems to dry, itchy skin.

You Get More Toxic Exposure from Taking a Chlorinated Water Shower Than From Drinking the Same Water!

Two of the very highly toxic and volatile chemicals, trichloroethylene and chloroform, have been proven as toxic contaminants found in most all municipal drinking water supplies. The National Academy of Sciences recently has estimated that hundreds of people die in the United States each year from the cancers caused largely by ingesting water pollutants from inhalation as air pollutants in the home. Inhalation exposure to water pollutants is largely ignored. Recent shocking data indicates that hot showers can liberate about 50% of the chloroform and 80% of the trichloroethylene into the air.

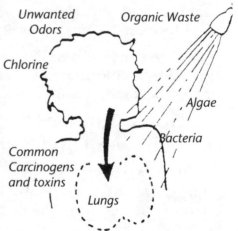

Tests show your body can absorb more toxic chlorine from a 10-minute shower than drinking 8 glasses of the same water. How can that be? A warm shower opens up your pores, causing your skin to act like a sponge. As a result, you not only inhale the toxic chlorine vapors, you absorb them through your skin, directly into your bloodstream – at a rate that is up to 6 times higher than drinking it.

In terms of cumulative damage to your health, showering in chlorinated water is one of the most dangerous risks you take daily. Short-term risks include: eyes, sinus, throat, skin and lung irritation. Long-term risks include: excessive free radical formation (that ages you!) higher vulnerability to genetic mutation and cancer development; and difficulty metabolizing cholesterol, causing hardened arteries. – Science News

The treatment of diseases should go to the root cause, and most often it is found in severe dehydration from lack of sufficient pure, distilled water, plus an unhealthy lifestyle!

Comparison of Water Treatment Methods
Steam Distilled Water is the Best

POLLUTANT	Filter Sediment	Filter Carbon	Deionization	Reverse Osmosis	Steam Distillation
Arsenic	○	○	●	●	●
Bacteria	○	○	○	◑	●
Cadmium	○	○	●	●	●
Calcium	○	○	●	●	●
Chlorides	○	○	●	●	●
Chlorine	○	●	○	●[1]	●[1]
Cryptosporidium	○	○	○	●	●
Detergents	○	◑	●	●	●
Fluorides	○	○	●	●	●
Lead	○	○	●	●	●
Magnesium	○	○	●	●	●
Nitrate	○	○	◑	◑	●
Organics	○	●	○	●[1]	●[1]
Pesticides	○	●	○	●[1]	●[1]
Phosphates	○	○	●	●	●
Radon	○	○	●	●	●
Sediment	●	◑	●	●	●
Sodium	○	○	●	●	●
Sulfates	○	◑	●	●	●
Viruses	○	○	○	○	●

○ Ineffective or No Reduction   ◑ Significant Reduction   ● Complete or Significant Reduction

1 – A Carbon Filter Needed (The best home distillers have also carbon filters.)

For info on reasonable water distillers & shower head filters for your home that remove harmful chemicals from your water call (800) 446-1990

113

Allergies, Daily Journal & Dr. Coca's Pulse Test

Almost every known food may cause some allergic reaction at times. Thus, foods used in "elimination" diets may cause allergic reactions in some individuals. Some are listed among the *Most Common Food Allergies*. Since reaction to these foods is generally low, they are widely used in making test diets. By keeping a food journal and tracking your pulse rate after meals you will soon know your "problem" foods. Allergic foods cause pulse to go up. (Take base pulse before meals and then 30 minutes after meals. If it increases 6 to 8 beats per minute – check foods for allergies.) See web *http://members.aol.com/SynergyHN/allergy22b.html*

If your body has a reaction after eating some particular food, especially if it happens each time you eat that food, you may have an allergy. Some allergic reactions are: wheezing, sneezing, stuffy nose, nasal drip or mucus, dark circles or waterbags under eyes, headaches, feeling light-headed or dizzy, fast heart beat, stomach or chest pains, diarrhea, extreme thirst, breaking out in a rash, swelling of extremities or stomach bloating, etc. (Read Dr. Arthur Coca's book, *The Pulse Test*.)

If you know what you're allergic to, you are lucky; if you don't, you had better find out as fast as possible and eliminate all irritating foods from your diet. To re-evaluate your daily life and have a health guide to your future, start a daily journal (8½ x 11 notebook) of foods eaten, pulse rate before and after meals, your reactions, moods, energy levels (ups/downs), weight, elimination and sleep patterns. You will discover the foods and situations causing problems. By charting your diet you will be amazed at the effects of eating certain foods. My dad kept his journal for over 70 years.

If you are hypersensitive to certain foods, you must reject them from your diet! There are hundreds of allergies and of course it is impossible here to take up each one. Many who suffer from this unpleasant affliction have allergies to milk, wheat, or some persons are allergic to all grains. Your journal helps you discover and accurately pinpoint the foods and situations causing problems. Start your journal today!

Most Common Food Allergies

- *MILK: Butter, Cheese, Cottage Cheese, Ice Cream, Milk, Yogurt, etc.*
- *CEREALS & GRAINS: Wheat, Corn, Buckwheat, Oats, Rye*
- *EGGS: Cakes, Custards, Dressings, Mayonnaise, Noodles*
- *FISH: Shellfish, Crabs, Lobster, Shrimp, Shadroe*
- *MEATS: Bacon, Chicken, Pork, Sausage, Veal, Smoked Products*
- *FRUITS: Citrus Fruits, Melons, Strawberries*
- *NUTS: Peanuts, Pecans, Walnuts, chemically dried preserved nuts*
- *MISCELLANEOUS: Chocolate, China Tea, Cocoa, Coffee, MSG, Palm and Cottonseed Oils, Salt, Spices and allergic reactions often caused by toxic pesticides on salad greens, vegetables, fruits, etc.*

Your Body Constantly Works for You – And You Must Work for Your Body!

The body is constantly breaking down old bone and tissue cells and replacing them with new ones. As the body casts off old minerals and broken-down cells, it must obtain fresh food supplies of essential elements for new cells. Scientists are only now beginning to understand that various kinds of dental problems, different types of arthritis and even some forms of artery hardening are due to body imbalances of calcium, phosphorus and magnesium. Many disorders can be caused by imbalances in the ratios of minerals to each other.

Each individual's healthy body requires a proper balance within itself of all the nutritive elements. It is just as bad for any individual to have too much of one item as it is to have too little of another one. For instance, it takes appropriate levels of phosphorus and magnesium to keep calcium in solution so it can be formed into new cells of bone and teeth. Yet there must not be too much magnesium nor too little calcium in the diet or old bone will be taken away and new bone will not be formed. We know that diets that are unbalanced can deplete the body of essential minerals and elements.

Diets high in meats, fish, eggs, grains and nuts or their products may provide unbalanced excesses of phosphorus which will leech calcium and magnesium from the bones, causing them to be lost in the urine.

A diet high in fats will tend to increase the intake of phosphorus from the intestines relative to calcium and other basic minerals. Such diets can also produce a loss of the body's basic minerals in the same way a high phosphorus diet does. Diets excessively high in fruits or their juices may provide unbalanced excesses of fruit sugars and of potassium in the body, which also can leech calcium and magnesium from the body.

115

When reading labels on products, you must be aware of added sodium content. Watch for the words "soda" and "sodium" and symbol "NA", these products contain sodium compounds. Some prescription drugs even contain large amounts of soduim.

Studies show that athletes tend to have high HDL (good cholesterol) levels.

Magnesium & Calcium Vital to Heart

Deficiencies of calcium and magnesium can produce all kinds of problems in the body – ranging from heart problems, dental decay and osteoporosis to muscular cramping, hyperactivity, muscular twitches, poor sleep patterns and also excessive frequency or uncontrolled urination patterns. Also, other mineral deficiencies or imbalances can cause health problems.

Therefore it's important to clean and detoxify the body by fasting and drinking only distilled, pure water or the juices of healthy organically grown vegetables and fruits. It's also important to provide the body with adequate sources of new minerals. This can be done by eating a diverse diet of organic vegetables that also includes kelp and other sea vegetables. Rice, soy and almond milks are good healthy alternatives to unhealthy cow's milk for babies and adults. See web: *notmilk.com*

Despite dietary sources as these, many adults and children living in so-called civilized cultures have low levels of essential minerals in their bodies. This is due to leeching caused by coffee, tea, cola, carbonated beverages and the ravages of long-term bad diets containing refined sugars, toxic aspartame and other sweets, as well as junk fast foods made from refined flours and foods containing high fat, high sugar, high salt and high cholesterol foods.

Additionally, the body's organ systems can be thrown out of balance by continued stress, toxins in our food, water and air, also by disease-produced injuries and by prenatal deficiencies arising from the mother's diet or lifestyle. The final result is that many people in our modern world need to take natural mineral supplements, as well as natural broad range multiple-vitamins.

Homeostasis and the Heart

Nutrition is important in the functions of the heart. A good diet, low in saturated fats, cholesterol and sodium, plus a sound nutritional program, supported by good exercise, work well together for the health of the heart and body. This can assist the body in maintaining homeostasis. Homeostasis (*homeo*=same; *stasis*=standing still) is defined as balance and harmony within the body.

Chapter 12

Doctor Healthy Foods

Importance of Balanced Body Chemistry

In this Heart Fitness Program we have thus far been emphasizing the *don'ts* because we consider these much more difficult to follow than the *do's*. Now we'll detail what kind of food program you should follow for heart fitness, health and longer life.

Every time you plan a meal, check off these four items on the fingers of your hand to see if you are eating a *nutritionally well-balanced combination of foods: protein, carbohydrates, fats, fruits and vegetables.*

1 Protein – Building Blocks of the Body

Protein foods are nuts, seeds (such as sunflower, sesame, pumpkin), nutritional yeast, wheat germ, soy beans, dairy products, whole grain cereals, meat, fish, poultry and protein supplements.

117

Protein is one of the most important food elements and *is essential for keeping the heart fit*. You must have protein for building every cell of your body. This fundamental demand of Mother Nature rules every creature living on the face of the Earth.

Protein is you – flesh, muscle, blood, heart, bones, skin and hair – all the components of the body are essentially composed of protein. *You are literally "built" of protein.* This basic function of your body – of converting food into living tissue – is one of life's miracles. Your life processes and the factors that help you resist disease are all composed of protein (amino acids) components.

Every time you move a muscle, every time your heart beats, every time you breathe, you consume protein in the form of amino acids. The link between protein and body tissue is the amino acids – and the bloodstream carries them to every part of the body where they work to repair, rebuild and maintain body tissues. They enrich blood and *condition* the organs, including the heart.

*It's magnificent to live long if one keeps
healthy, alert, youthful and active. – Harry Fosdick*

Amino Acids – The Body's Building Blocks

Human tissue is renewed daily. Scientists once believed that there were great masses of protein in the body in an inactive state – stores of protein built up in the muscles, tissues and organs which remain there until the body might need them. Now we know that the great builder protein is not stationary, but in motion. This activity requires a replenishment of essential protein for the rebuilding process, especially in older people.

What is the connection between Amino Acids and proteins? Amino Acids are the building blocks from which different food proteins are constructed. When we eat a protein food, such as meat or soybeans, the natural hydrochloric acid in the stomach *digests* the protein, releasing the Aminos Acids. They are the link between the food we eat and assimilate for our body's tissues. Amino Acids are what makes our food turn into us!

Unlike vitamins, the *activators* in our nutrition, Amino Acids actually enter into the structure of the body tissue itself. They are the very foundation of all protein foods. They build muscles, tissues and organs and circulate freely in the blood – the body's vital lifestream. Your blood is your precious river of life – protect it!

The phytochemicals found in soy are specifically known as isoflavins. These isoflavins have been shown to be strong antioxidents that help repair cellular damage in the body, and they have anti-tumor effects. Soy can contribute to optimal health and has remarkable health-promoting properties. See phytochemical chart on page 145.

Amino Acids – Life-Givers & Life-Extenders

Famous Pioneer Endocrinologist and Biochemist, Dr. W. Donner Denckla, with the National Institute of Health, has been immersed in pathfinding research on longevity for years. Dr. Denckla has the opinion that ageing is not inevitable and that Amino Acids and their interaction with a hormone secreted by the pituitary gland seem to be the key to slowing down ageing.

The longevity secret is eating & drinking intelligently. – Gayelord Hauser

If we could look within the body, we would see all the living cells that make up the tissues, organs and bloodstream are in a highly active state. Paul C. Bragg was the first to preach the gospel of Amino Acids, their relationship to ageing and how they can help keep you younger, longer! He stressed that when the protein supply – the Amino Acids – are replenished regularly, the new cells that are constantly growing and being born can then thrive and live with more positive intensity! Another important benefit of Amino Acids – they help form antibodies to fight germs, infections and disease!

Bragg Introduces Miracles of Soybeans

Over 88 years ago my father introduced Bragg Liquid Aminos to the health-minded as a way to help them increase natural, life-building vegetable protein intake in a form that's easily digestible and delicious to use! It's a liquid form of soy protein from pure, healthy (certified non-genetically engineered) soybeans – a 100% health product that contains no coloring agents, preservatives or added sodium. Lack of adequate Amino Acids in your body may make it impossible for the vitamins and minerals to perform their specific duties. Amino Acids are inseparably interwoven with vitamins and minerals for good sound nutrition. Bragg Liquid Aminos contains no meat, and adds delicious natural flavors and zest to most all foods by sprinkling or spraying on foods. It's the most delicious, nutritious and unique gourmet health seasoning, for it contains 16 important vital Amino Acids and Isoflavins for super health.

What are Amino Acids? They're the building blocks of all our organs and tissues. They are the building blocks of proteins. They are essential for production of energy within ourselves, for detoxification and for the vital transmission of nerve impulses. In short, they are the very soup of life, and they are almost always overlooked and neglected. – H. J. Hoegerman, M.D.

Amino Acids are needed for building every part of the body . . . bones, blood, hair, skin, nails and glands – and are Mother Nature's and God's life–giving secret to a long, vital life. – Paul C. Bragg

Up to 90% of deaths annually are self-inflicted by an unhealthy lifestyle!

2 | Carbohydrates – Starches and Sugars

Starches and sugars come under the classification, carbohydrates, in the FDA standard for food groups. These provide the principle source of food energy. Carbohydrates are needed as fuel for muscular work and physical activity. Excess sugars and starches that are not utilized as energy are transformed by the body chemistry into fat and stored in the least active body parts.

Carbohydrates originate in plants as sugars created by photosynthesis. Then they are formed into clusters as starches. Consumed by humans, they are broken down by the body's metabolism into a simple sugar – glucose – for use by the cells of the body. It is important that you eat only natural starches and sugars, and avoid those which are refined and depleted of vital elements (refined white flour, sugar and their refined products, etc.).

Natural starches and some natural sugars are found in all fresh fruits and vegetables, honey, pure maple syrup, sorghum, stevia and blackstrap molasses, organic whole grains and their flours (wheat, oats, rye, etc.), beans, lentils and peas, organic brown rice and potatoes. In fact, all natural foods contain some carbohydrates.

3 | Fats Can Be Healthy or Unhealthy

Fat is also an important source of dietary energy. It has more than twice the energy value of the same amount of carbohydrates or protein. As already pointed out elsewhere in our Heart Fitness Program, a certain amount of fat and even cholesterol is part of a healthy diet. Let us remind you that your fat intake should ideally consist of only unsaturated fats. The saturated fats in meat, eggs, poultry and dairy products should be avoided or kept to a minimum. It is these saturated fats which can overload your body with cholesterol.

Cholesterol is a fatty substance produced daily by the liver for normal use in the body. As noted earlier, when we overload our bloodstream with cholesterol (saturated fats) in our diet, it can stockpile and form waxy deposits on artery walls and block blood flow.

Let food be your medicine, and medicine be your food. – Hippocrates

The Function of Fat in the Body

Our nerves, muscles and organs must be *cushioned* by a normal amount of fat. If we did not have a certain amount of fat in our *gluteus maximus* (the buttocks), for example, we would never be able to sit down because we would have to sit directly on our muscles and bones.

Those who wish to lose weight should reduce the *bad, saturated fat* content of their diet, and those who wish to gain should increase their *good, unsaturated fat* intake. But even when on a reducing diet, there should be some fat in your diet because it plays an important and essential role in your body's chemistry.

Stored in the body, fat provides a source of heat and energy, while the accumulation of a certain amount of fat around the vital organs (such as the kidneys) gives great protection against cold and injury.

Fat also has a function to perform in the body's cells, for which special fats known as unsaturated fatty acids are needed in small amounts. Without these a roughness or scaliness of the skin would result.

Fats have another all-important function: they carry the fat-soluble vitamins A, D, E and K through the body.

As you can see, a certain amount of fat in the diet is necessary to a healthy functioning body. But it's the kind of fat that is most important! Unsaturated fat is best. Caution – go light on clogging saturated fats!

Low Fat Meals Cut Heart Disease Risk

A British research report by Dr. George Miller of Britain's Medical Research Council stated: *High fat meals make the blood more prone to clot within 6 to 7 hours after eating. Low fat meals can almost immediately reverse this condition. Most heart attacks occur in the early morning. One reason may be the overnight clotting effects of a high fat dinner. Researchers feel that by cutting fats from your diet, you may be able to add years to your life and cut the risk of heart disease!* Also the recent University of Chicago scientific research supports Dr. Miller's landmark statement that the healthiest meals for the heart are the low-fat, vegetarian diets with ample fruits and vegetables.

- Remember, meat-free and dairy-free is healthiest.
- Spend most of your time in the produce department.
- Try new varieties of produce. Look at those with the most intense colors and remember organic is best!
- Don't forget about pasta made from whole-grains.
- Go straight for the whole-grain breads section.
- Buy unrefined, low-fat, sugarless, high-fiber cereals.
- When buying packaged, canned, frozen foods – read labels.
- Don't underestimate beans – whether dried, frozen or canned they are delicious and healthy for you.
- Buy low- or no-fat snacks – there are many choices. Careful, some are high in salt, sugar and calories.
- Replace milk and low-fat dairy products with soy, nut and rice milks, and soy and tofu cheeses, etc.

In 1998, the world lost one of its beloved, strong and dedicated health crusaders. Dr. Charles Raymond Attwood was a devoted pediatrician for over 35 years. He championed a low-fat vegetarian menu for children, was a strong health and nutrition activist and an associate of Dr. Benjamin Spock. *www.vegsource.com*

Dr. Charles Attwood – Great Health Crusader

As a doctor, humanitarian and Fellow of the American Academy of Pediatrics, Dr. Attwood fought many battles against mainstream medicine and big business to ensure the health of people everywhere, particularly children. One major battle occurred in 1996. As a member of the Center for Science in the Public Interest, Dr. Attwood led opposition to the giant Gerber Baby Food Company's practice of diluting its baby foods with water, sugar and starch. He won! Gerber stopped this 40 year crime against America's children. Now their foods are 100% fruits and vegetables. Other baby food companies then followed.

In the last 20 years, Dr. Attwood held high the banner advocating a low-fat, plant-based diet as the most healthy for youngsters. His highly praised 1995 book, *Low-fat Prescription for Kids* makes a strong scientific argument for this kind of diet. His research shows in order to avoid the leading causes of premature death later as adults, namely: heart disease, stroke, cancers, diabetes, etc. it's important children follow his program.

Raw Nuts and Seeds Are Good Food

Gary Null, a leading health activist writes in his book, *The Complete Guide to Sensible Eating, Raw nuts and seeds are fine sources of protein, minerals (especially magnesium), some B vitamins and unsaturated fatty acids. Delicious as snack foods or used with other foods.* www.garynull.com

There are few foods that are more highly packed with life force than raw seeds and nuts. Consider the Japanese archaeologist who found millet-like seeds in an ancient tomb in Egypt which had lain dormant in the dark for 4,000 years. He put them in some water and they sprouted! There are more than 300 kinds of seeds and nuts that grow around the world and they vary nutritionally, but most of them are good sources of B vitamins, (thiamine and folate) and iron, magnesuim and zinc. Many of them are also loaded with vitamin E, protein and fiber. Raw nuts and seeds, as a snack food (try this great combo – nuts and raisins) are excelled by no other food, supplying the body with healthy polyunsaturuated fats, protein and nutrients it needs for heart health and good nutrition.

123

To make Nut Butters: grind 1½ cups of raw unsalted nuts in a food processor or blender, turning the machine off every 20 seconds. Continue grinding nuts down until they're a thick, fudge-like paste. Then add sunflower or nut oil (start with 1 tablespoon and add more only if necessary), blend until smooth. Keep refrigerated.

The large network of veins and arteries through which your blood circulates, need to be open, clear and strong to keep your blood circulating. High blood pressure is a sign they are straining, having to squeeze extra hard to push your blood through. This wears them out and your heart, too. Change your lifestyle.

Strokes result when blood clots form in the arteries, blocking nutrients to brain cells. Omega 3 fish oils are anticoagulants present in fish such as tuna or salmon. You can also get a good dose in a daily teaspoon of flaxseed oil. Onions and garlic are other natural anticoagulants.

Automated External Defibrillator (AED) Offers Fast Miracle –

for victims of sudden cardiac arrest. A recent report in the New England Journal of Medicine states that the survival rate for those who received their first defibrillation no later than 3 minutes after a collapse was 74%, as opposed to 49% survival rate for those defibrillated after more than 3 minutes. The FAA has decided to have medium to large passenger planes carry an AED. Med centers, big businesses, universities, schools, cruise ships etc. soon will have one in their first aid kits for emergencies. www. nejm.org

Medtronic's LIFEPAK® 500 AED, portable • (800) 442-1142

Organic Virgin Olive Oil Highly Recommended

Mother Nature has provided us with wonderful healthy oils which can be used in preparing foods, mayonnaise and salad dressings or for sautéing and marinating, etc. Virgin, cold-pressed olive oil has been used for centuries. Even Hippocrates used olive oil in his practice (see page 152). Do try Bragg's Organic Extra Virgin (first pressed) Olive Oil – it's the healthiest of oils!

Other good oils are cold-pressed safflower, sesame, sunflower and soybean oils. These oils can be used in salad dressings, recipes, baking, etc. We still use oils sparingly. They're healthy in polyunsaturated and unsaturated fatty acids. Please, don't use genetically engineered canola oil.

Another favorite oil of ours is organic unrefined flaxseed oil which is the richest source of omega-3 essential fatty acids (more than double that of fish oils). We also use hempseed oil. These two fragile oils must be kept cold, preferably in the freezer (they do not solidify) and they should not be heated. You can add them to foods after they have been cooked. We suggest you add 1 to 2 teaspoons daily of these oils to your diet, for the omega fatty acids are vital to your bodily functions, especially the heart! (see page 146 for Pep Drink)

4 | Protective Foods – Fruits & Vegetables

Remember that we told you that three-fifths of your diet should consist of organic, raw and lightly cooked vegetables and fresh fruits. These foods not only contribute isoflavins, vitamins and organic minerals to the diet, but they also add the bulk and moisture required for healthy elimination and smooth body functioning. They also help maintain the alkaline reserve of the body and add variety, color, flavor and texture to the diet.

Vegetables are virtually fat-free and contain no cholesterol! The ideal way to get the full amount of vitamins and minerals from organic vegetables is in their raw state, in fresh vegetable salads or as garnishes with meals. When cooking vegetables some vitamins and minerals may be lost.

The nervousness and peevishness of our times are chiefly attributable to tea and coffee. – Dr. Bock, 1910

Fresh Juices Are Best

Freshly prepared organic vegetable and fruit juices are ideal ways to add vitamins and minerals to your diet. We enjoy carrot, celery and beet juice mixed together. See page 159 for more delicious combinations. There are two *Bragg Health Recipe Books* to choose from *(100% vegetarian and non-vegetarian)* that will be helpful in planning your health-building meals. Both have 100's of delicious recipes.

The Importance of Lecithin

The liver performs over five hundred separate jobs – one is producing the body's normal cholesterol and an important substance called lecithin. Lecithin is one of God's greatest gifts to man! It mixes with the bile in the gall bladder and is emptied along with the bile into the small intestine to help in the digestion of fats as they leave the stomach. Lecithin is a fat homogenizing agent which breaks up fat into tiny particles. One of the great health discoveries of Nutritional Science is the role of lecithin (from soybeans) and linoleic acid (from safflower oil) in helping the body to dispose of these excess fats. You can see that a deficiency of these two agents may cause serious coronary blockage problems.

The soybean is the richest source of lecithin. It's also found in all products which contain fat, such as the germ (part that sprouts) of various grains. Lecithin and wheat germ are very much alike in appearance. Commercial lecithin has a wide variety of uses. It is used to lubricate precision machines where oil needs to be spread thinly. It's also important in confectionery and baking businesses for its natural homogenizing effect.

When Dad was associate editor of Macfadden's *Physical Culture Magazine* – he was sent on an expedition into China – soybean's original home. For thousands of years the Chinese used soybeans. About 80% of their food is produced from soybeans in one form or another.

There is a high concentration of lecithin in heart cells and in the sheathing around the brain, spinal cord and nerves. Lecithin supplements come from the diversified, healthy soybean. Lecithin is a natural fat emulsifier and helps reduce larger dangerous LDL cholesterol globules and elevates smaller, healthier HDL particles and also increases vital choline levels.

To his amazement, he again found many people who were living unbelievably long lives, like Zora Agha of Turkey. It was not unusual to find men and women from 125 to 135 years of age. Among these people, heart attacks, strokes, paralysis, coronary thrombosis and degenerative artery diseases were practically unknown! Eating soybeans in various forms meant they got large amounts of lecithin in their simple diet. The lecithin homogenized (dissolved) their dietary fats. Thus their level of blood-fat or blood cholesterol remained normal.

Soybean Products for Healthy Heart & Nerves

We have been recommending the use of soybeans and its products to the health-conscious people of America since 1912. Lecithin – of which the soybean is the richest source – is not just important in the digestion of fats. The functioning of the nervous system and the glands are greatly aided by the phospholipids, one of the most important constituents of lecithin. That's why it's found in the nervous system and in every cell of the body. Nutritional Science teaches us that the nerves and cardiovascular system both require lecithin and the vitamin B-complex rich foods. (See pages 39, 153.)

Scientists have cited that breast cancer in Asian women is much lower than that in American women, largely due to the fact that Asian women consume a diet high in soy protein which contains Isoflavines. These Isoflavines also lower blood cholesterol levels (page 145) which is vitally important for a healthy heart!

What Are Live Foods?

Live foods are the living, vital foods for health and longevity and are perishable and some spoil quickly. We have been ignorant, foolish and almost idiotic in allowing our various foods to be so refined that the vital and essential elements that Mother Nature gave them are refined out of them. We are buying and eating the depleted, devitalized mess that remains. This refining of foods is destroying our health, hearts and bodies!

To work the head, temperance must be carried into the diet. – Beecher

Vitamin E & Raw Wheat Germ – Health Builders

Mother Nature invested raw wheat germ with one of the most valuable nutrients – vitamin E. And now it is coming to the aid of civilized man to help him regain the robust health he lost by eating devitalized foods.

Dr. Cureton of the University of Illinois, who is recognized as one of the greatest living authorities on internal and external physical fitness, recommends raw wheat germ (little yellowish flakes), wheat germ oil and vitamin E capsules. They are especially useful in providing a great boost for athletes and others who desire to be in the highest state of physical fitness. Athletic coaches all over the world are following this advice to get the best performance from their athletes. In our opinion *raw wheat germ (vacuum packed), wheat germ oil and Vitamin E should be part of the nutritional program of everyone* – not just athletes! Vitamin E capsules are also recommended as the oil is more protected from rancidity.

In the process of flour milling, refining removes the raw wheat germ to create white flour. Millers realize that wheat germ is a fragile, natural oil reservoir which will go rancid quickly. Commercial food requires a long shelf life. The average American demands that everything they buy never spoil. That is why so many American foods are refined and why over 700 chemicals and poisons are used to preserve them!

Breakfast Should Be An Occasional Meal

On rare mornings when we eat breakfast, we have organic whole grain cereal, oatmeal or cornmeal, a sliced banana over the cereal, with some honey, etc. and rice or soy milk. Make your own by combining tbsp of soy powder with ½ glass of water and ½ tsp vanilla or 100% maple syrup in a jar and shake. It's delicious and healthy!

A rich food source of vitamin E is cornmeal mush, made with organic stoneground yellow cornmeal (not the refined, dead, GMO, degerminated variety of corn found in most supermarkets). On the next pages are the Bragg family's favorite cornmeal recipe, plus a chart for making sure you get your vitamin E from the foods you eat.

Patricia's Organic Cornmeal Mush

1 cup organic yellow cornmeal (coarse ground best)
2½ cups distilled water   3 Tbsp raisins (optional)

Moisten cornmeal with ½ cup distilled water. Boil balance (2 cups) of water, then slowly add moistened cornmeal and raisins. Mix well. When evenly thickened, turn heat low and cook for 10 to 15 minutes. Serve hot. Top with honey, blackstrap molasses or 100% maple syrup (our favorite). Then, if desired, top with sliced bananas or organic fresh fruit and try some soy or rice milk.

NOTE: If you are serving this to one or two people, there might be some mush left. Pour it into a flat pan, let it cool, and store in refrigerator. For breakfast – or even a main meal – slice and dip in egg batter and roll in wheat germ. Lightly sauté in Bragg Olive Oil and serve plain, hot, or top with honey, blackstrap molasses or maple syrup.

Soy Tofu Scramble

128

2 cups firm tofu, crumbled
2 tsps Bragg Organic Olive Oil
⅛ tsp ground cumin
¼ tsp fresh garlic or powder

2 green onions, chopped
diced tomatoes (optional)
½ tsp Bragg Liquid Aminos
Pinch Italian herbs

In a wok, lightly sauté green onions in olive oil for 3 minutes, then add remaining ingredients and cook 3 to 5 minutes longer. You can add fresh diced tomatoes or other veggies. Serves 2 to 4.

Soy Tofu French Toast

½ lb tofu (soft)
¼ tsp nutmeg

⅓ tsp cinnamon powder
1 Tbsp honey

Blend tofu with enough water (distilled) to make a slightly runny batter. Dip whole grain bread slices in batter and sauté until brown in a little soy oil or butter. Turn over and cook the other side. Serve hot with honey or pure maple syrup. Serves 2.

Or, for variety, the Bragg family likes to have an occasional breakfast of steel-cut organic oats, cooked with raisins or sun-dried apricots, served with sliced bananas and 100% maple syrup. Yummy!

High sugar consumption can overstimulate your whole system, and too much sugar can lead to many problems, ranging from obesity, heart trouble, poor circulation to high blood sugar levels and diabetes.

Vitamin E-Rich Healthy Foods Are Important for Healthy Hearts

This is a list of healthy foods that contain the following notable amounts of precious vitamin E. This list was compiled from *Bridges Food and Beverage Analyses*. Buy organic sources – they are best.

Food	Quantity	Vitamin E IU's
Apples	1 medium	0.74
Bananas	1 medium	0.40
Barley	½ cup	4.20
Beans, navy	½ cup	3.60
Butter (salt-free)	6 tablespoons	2.40
Carrots	1 cup	0.45
Celery, green	½ cup	2.60
Corn, dried for popcorn	1 cup	20.00
Cornmeal, yellow	½ cup	1.70
Corn oil	6 tablespoons	87.00
Eggs, fertile	2	2.00
Endive, escarole	½ cup	2.00
Flour, whole grain	1 cup	54.00
Grapefruit	½	0.52
Kale	½ cup	8.00
Lettuce	6 leaves	0.50
Oatmeal	½ cup	2.00
Olive Oil (virgin)	½ cup	5.00
Onions, raw	2 medium	0.26
Oranges	1 small	0.24
Parsley	½ cup	5.50
Peas, green	1 cup	4.00
Potatoes, white	1 medium	0.06
Potatoes, sweet	1 small	4.00
Rice, brown	1 cup cooked	2.40
Rye	½ cup	3.00
Soybean Oil	6 tablespoons	140.00
Sunflower Seeds, raw	½ cup	31.00
Wheat Germ Oil	6 tablespoons	50 – 420.00

The Bragg Gourmet Health Recipe Book (448 pages) –
1,000 Delicious, Healthy Recipes
See back pages for book list.

Vitamin E is a dynamic weapon against wrinkles and ageing. – Prevention Magazine

A recent revealing study of nurses whose daily vitamin E intake was 100 mgs and more had a 36% lower risk of heart attack and 23% lower risk of stroke.

Calcium is Important for a Fit Heart

Consider the shocking fact that 85% of Americans are deficient in calcium! Most people associate calcium with the teeth and bones, which is correct since a deficiency of this important mineral will lead to the deterioration of these hard tissues. Calcium is also very important for the nerves of the body and many people suffer leg cramps as a result of a calcium deficiency. Calcium also plays a very needed, important role in the functioning of the human heart. Calcium is a natural constituent of the material that causes the blood to clot. If we did not have calcium in our bloodstream, we could prick a finger with a needle and bleed to death!

Every few minutes the heart is bathed by the calcium of the body chemistry. It is a crucial component in the activity of a healthy heart. Being the most powerful muscle in the entire body, the heart requires adequate calcium for its efficient functioning. Be good to your heart and maintain a good calcium balance. Study calcium chart.

Milk is Not a Good Source of Calcium

Nearly everyone has the idea that the problem of calcium deficiency will be solved if they just drink milk. This is not completely true. In the first place, practically all the milk in the U.S. is pasteurized, which robs and greatly reduces the availability of the milk's calcium.

Dr. Harold D. Lynch – famous author, researcher and physician – said recently **almost fanatic use of milk as a beverage has added more complications than benefits to child nutrition.** He further states **milk may often be a primary cause of poor nutrition in children!**

This might be due to the fact that proportionate amounts of Vitamins A and D and phosphorus must be present in the metabolism for the proper absorption and utilization of calcium by the body; another reason why proper nutrition and a balanced diet are so important!

Whole milk is a carrier of large amounts of saturated fat (cholesterol) and can lead to atherosclerosis. This food is just for cow's babies. It's not for humans if they wish to maintain a healthy heart for a long life!

Benefit From Natural Foods Rich in Calcium

There are some very fine sources of calcium other than milk. Scientists feel raw bonemeal is one of the best, as well as eggshell calcium, oyster shell calcium and bone marrow calcium. We prefer the calcium found in kale, corn, beans, veggies and soy tofu. In fact, as Dr. Lynch and Dr. Neal Barnard point out, all natural foods contain appreciable amounts of calcium. This chart shows some of the many foods that contain large amounts of calcium you should include in your diet.

Calcium Content of Some Common Foods

Food Source	mgs	Food Source	mgs
Almonds, 1 oz	80	Kale, (steamed) 1C	180
Artichokes, (steamed) 1C	51	Kohlrabi, (steamed) 1C	40
Beans, (kidney, pinto, red) 1 C	89	Mustard greens, 1C	138
Beans, (great northern, navy) 1C	128	Oatmeal, 1C	120
Beans, (white) 1C	161	Orange, 1 large	96
Blackstrap molasses, 1 Tbsp	137	Prunes, 4 whole	45
Bok choy, (steamed) 1C	158	Raisins, 4 oz.	45
Broccoli, (steamed) 1C	178	Rhubarb, (cooked) 1C	105
Brussel sprouts, (steamed) 1C	56	Rutabaga, (steamed) 1C	72
Buckwheat pancake, 1	99	Sesame seeds (unhulled) 1 oz	381
Cabbage, (steamed) 1C	50	Spinach (steamed) 1C	244
Cauliflower, (steamed) 1C	34	Soybeans, 1 C	73
Collards, (steamed) 1C	152	Soymilk, fortified	150
Corn tortilla	60	Tofu, firm ½ C	258
Cornbread, 1 piece	28	Turnip greens, 1C	198
Figs, (5 medium)	135	Whole wheat bread, 1 slice	17

Sources: *Back to Eden,* Jethro Kloss; *Health Nutrient Bible,* Lynne Sonberg; website: veggiepower.ca/caltable.htm, chart by Brenda Davis, R.D.

Read these 2 important books on milk and why to avoid milk:
- Mad Cows and Milk Gate *by Virgil Hulse M.D. (541) 482-2048*
- Milk, the Deadly Poison *by Robert Cohen (888) 668-6455*

Also visit these important websites:
- notmilk.com and • milkgate.com

The human body has one ability not possessed by any machine – the body has the ability to repair itself. – George W. Crile

---

The World Health Organization reported recently that 24.5 million people worldwide – nearly 50% of the yearly deaths – are victims of just 3 chronic conditions linked to unhealthy lifestyles: circulatory diseases (especially heart attacks and strokes), cancer and lung disease! – US News and World Report

The Deadly Truth About Salt

For centuries, the expression *the salt of the earth* has been used as a catch-all phrase to describe something as good and essential. Yet nothing could be more wrong. That *harmless* product that you shake on top of your food every day may actually bury you!

Consider these startling facts on salt:

1. **Salt is not a food!** There is no more justification for its culinary use than there is for potassium chloride, calcium chloride, barium chloride or any other harmful chemical that is used as a food seasoning.

2. **Salt cannot be digested, assimilated or utilized by the body.** Salt has no nutritional value! It has no vitamins! No organic minerals! No nutrients of any kind! Instead, it is positively harmful and can cause trouble in the kidneys, bladder, heart, arteries, veins and blood vessels. Salt may waterlog the tissues, causing water retention.

3. **Salt may act as a heart poison.** It also increases the irritability of the nervous system and the body.

4. **Salt robs calcium from the body** and attacks the mucus lining throughout the gastrointestinal tract.

The Myth of the "Salt Lick"

Is a low-salt diet a nutritionally deficient diet? Don't we need plenty of salt in our diets to keep us in top physical condition? This is a popular notion, but is it true? People will tell you that animals will travel for miles to visit so-called *salt licks*. My father investigated the salt licks where wild forest animals congregated for miles around to lick the soil. The one chemical property all of these sites commonly known as *salt licks* had in common was *complete absence of sodium chloride (common salt)!* There was absolutely no organic or inorganic sodium at the salt licks! *But theses soils had an abundance of organic minerals and nutrients which the animals naturally craved.*

It's a little known fact that about 80% of sodium we eat comes not from salt we add at the table or during cooking, but from processed, packaged foods.
– Tufts University Nutrition Letter

Salt Affects Your Blood Pressure

What causes high blood pressure? Medical Science recognizes many causes: tension, strains, stress, toxic substances such as cigarettes and gasoline, food additives, insecticide sprays, etc. and the side effects of drugs and industrial toxins are all suspect. What can you do to protect yourself from these injurious agents? You would do well to exclude as many of these harmful factors from your environment and life as soon as possible!

However, there is one cause of high blood pressure which can be easily avoided. *Sodium chloride (common table salt) is the major cause of high blood pressure!* Up to now, we have been talking about causing high blood pressure in the *normal* person. But how about the effects of salt on those millions suffering from our country's most prevalent and preventable ailment – excess weight? This is a prime area for research because obesity is known to be frequently accompanied by high blood pressure. Medical researchers proclaim a link between high blood pressure and salt intake in obesity.

133

Salt is Not Essential to Life

It is frequently claimed that salt is essential for life. However, there is no scientific basis to this belief. The truth is that entire primitive populations today use absolutely no salt and have never used it (most have no arthritis, cancer, etc.). If salt were essential to life, these people would have disappeared long ago. The proof salt is not needed is they are not only alive, but have better health than most Americans! Seems the *false necessity* of salt is mostly a money-making, harmful product.

Salt is Not Necessary to Combat Heat

There has been a great deal of propaganda in recent years about using salt in hot weather. The claim is made that the body loses a great deal of salt via perspiration and that this loss must be compensated for by consuming additional amounts of salt. Otherwise, according to this theory, great weakness and inability to continue normal activities will result. Hence factory workers are advised to take salt tablets in hot weather. We have watched many factory workers take these salt tablets, and we have also seen many of them become quite ill afterward. In fact, toxic reactions frequently follow the use of salt tablets. Vomiting and indigestion appear to be the 2 most common side effects and – as far as enabling one to stand the heat better is concerned – these dangerous supplements have no effect.

Death Valley Hike Proved Salt Dangerous

To prove definitely to my dad that he did not need salt during extremely hot weather, he went to Death Valley, California, one of the hottest spots in the entire world during July and August. On his first test he hired 10 husky young college athletes to make the hike in Death Valley from Furnace Creek Ranch to Stovepipe Wells, a distance of approximately 30 miles.

The boys had salt tablets and all the water they could drink . . . and a station wagon filled with plenty of food that contained salty foods like bread, buns, crackers, cheese, luncheon meats and hot dogs. They each ate, drank and took as many salt tablets as they desired. Dad had no salt and fasted during the 30 mile hike. They began the hike on a sweltering July morning. The higher the sun rose, the hotter it became! Up went the heat until at noon it stood at 130 degrees – a dry, hot heat that seemed to want to melt and defeat these hikers!

The college boys gobbled the salt tablets and guzzled quarts of cool water. For lunch they drank cola drinks with ham and cheese sandwiches. They rested a half hour after lunch and then continued their rugged hike across the red hot blazing sands. Soon things were beginning to happen to those strong, husky college boys.

First, 3 of them got violently ill and threw up all they ate and drank for lunch. They got dizzy, turned deathly pale and weakness overcame them. They quit the hike immediately and were driven back to the Furnace Creek Ranch. The hike went on with 7 college athletes continuing.

The desire for salty foods is an acquired taste. Your tastebuds can be retrained to appreciate the true flavors of foods. – Neal Barnard, M.D., *Food for Life.*

Bragg - the Only Non-Salt User Finished Hike

As the hike progressed, the athletes drank large amounts of cold water and took more salt tablets. Then suddenly 5 of them got stomach cramps and became deathly ill. Up came the water and their lunch. These 5 had to be driven back. That left but 2 out of 10 hikers. It was now about 4 pm and the merciless sun beat down on them with great fury. Almost on the hour, the last remaining salt tablet-eating athlete collapsed under that hot sun and was rushed back for medical care.

That left only my dad on the test and he felt great! He was not full of salt tablets nor food because he was on a fast. The college boys wanted cold water, but Dad drank only unchilled, pure distilled water. He finished the 30 mile hike in good time and had no ill effects whatsoever! He camped out for the night. The next day he arose, and on distilled water only, hiked another 30 miles back to the ranch without food or salt tablets. The doctors examined him and found him to be in excellent physical condition with no ill affects from the hot climate and the strenuous hike.

135

Break the Deadly Salt Habit!

In our expeditions over the world we have met many primitive tribes in the tropics that use no salt. And while they are not bothered by the heat, salt-eating white people invariably complain about the hot weather. This seems to indicate that some commercial motive lies behind the *eat more salt in hot weather* campaign.

People undoubtedly would not add inorganic salt to their food if they were never taught to do so in the first place. *The taste for salt is an acquired one.* The craving for salt ceases a short time after it is eliminated from the diet. It is only during the first few weeks after the use of table salt is discontinued that it is really missed. After the initial period of abstinence there is little difficulty. In fact, many of our health students who have broken the deadly salt habit write us to say that now they cannot stand salted foods! When someone serves them salted foods, it gives them an abnormal thirst for liquids!

What Table Salt Does to Your Stomach

An important objection to table salt is the fact that it *interferes with the normal digestion of food*. Pepsin, an enzyme found in the hydrochloric acid of the stomach, is essential for the digestion of proteins. Only 50% as much pepsin is secreted as would otherwise be the case when salt is used. Obviously the digestion of protein foods will be incomplete or too slow under such conditions. The results are excessive putrefaction of protein, bloating, gas and digestive distress, which effects millions.

Sea Kelp is an Excellent Salt Substitute
It's a Tasty, Healthy, Organic Sodium

Many outstanding heart specialists heartily endorse a no-salt diet. There are some excellent seasoning substitutes available to satisfy an acquired craving for salt. In the Bragg home we use sea kelp granulars, herbs, garlic, vegetable seasonings and Bragg Liquid Aminos.

In our opinion, sea kelp is an ideal salt substitute. It gives all foods – salads, vegetables, etc. – a tangy taste as Bragg Aminos does. The Bragg Products and sea kelp granulars (rich in folate, calcium & magnesium to build new blood cells) are available at health food stores. Fresh and powdered garlic, lemon juice and Braggs organic, raw apple cider vinegar are excellent seasoners, also, Italian and French herbs add delicious flavors to foods.

Take a lesson from world famous French chefs! The marvelous flavor of French dishes is achieved by the skillful use of garlic, onions, mushrooms, herbs – not with salt! French cooking is called *rich* – but it's a richness of taste and not of content. The best French chefs use very little fat and most use no salt at all!

The American Heart Association says that daily sodium intake should be less than 2,400 milligrams per day, which is about 1¼ teaspoons of sodium chloride (table salt –inorganic sodium). We recommend using NO table salt. Throwing away the salt shaker is a positive step towards living The Bragg Healthy Lifestyle! Get your natural organic sodium from natural healthy foods.

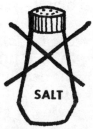

SALT

Natural Foods Have Organic Sodium

Organic sodium is one of the 16 minerals that are *required for perfect mineral balance* in the human body. Absorbable sodium is the most plentiful organic mineral found in all fresh fruits and vegetables, *especially beets, celery and stringbeans*. Be assured that when you eat a balanced diet of plant-based natural foods you will receive sufficient organic sodium. Again let us tell you that you must *put down that salt shaker and not pick it up again,* if you want a powerful, long-lasting heart!

Your Educated Taste Buds will Guide You

After you give up salt you will appreciate the natural flavor of foods. Dad was reared in the South where salt was used plentifully to season nearly all foods. His 260 taste buds were conditioned to the heavy taste of salt. At 16 he was a victim of tuberculosis. After three American Sanitoriums and no improvement, his mother took him to a *Natural TB Sanitorium* in the Swiss Alps where they were against salt in the diet, something new to Dad! His health returned miraculously. (His body was cleansed and healed – nature's way for a miracle recovery.)

At first, Dad's taste buds rebelled. But no salt was permitted – so he re-educated his taste buds to a saltless diet. Any bad habit is difficult to overcome at first and the salt habit surely had Dad in its clutches, as it has millions of Americans! But once his taste buds learned the difference, he started to taste and enjoy the real, natural flavors of food for the first time in his life.

Some health-minded people use *sea salt* rather than *table (land) salt*. There's little difference between these two! They are *both inorganic* and *loaded with sodium chloride!* Your 260 taste buds will guide you after you have discarded salt, for they will become very keen and sensitive and will reject salty foods. You will begin to enjoy tasting all the delicious flavors of natural foods.

The seat of knowledge is in the head; of wisdom, in the heart. We are sure to judge wrong if we do not feel right. – William Hazlit

Eliminating Meat is Safer and Healthier!

Most uninformed nutritionists call meat the #1 source of protein. Those proteins coming from the vegetable kingdom are referred to as the #2 proteins. This is a sad and terrible mistake. It should be the other way around! Because in this day and age, almost all meat is laden with herbicides, fungicides, pesticides and other chemicals that are sprayed on or poured into the feed which these animals consume. They are also pumped full of growth hormones, antibiotics and all kinds of drugs to fatten them up and keep them from dying from the extremely unhealthy conditions most of them live in! Many of them are forced-fed the dead, ground up carcasses of other feed lot animals who, for a variety of sad reasons, didn't make it to the slaughterhouse.

The chemical reaction from fear is adrenaline! Fear is caused when a choke chain is around the neck of cattle to keep them in line. It's then shoved onto a conveyor belt and beheaded like those in front of them. Unused adrenaline is extremely toxic. Most of the meat that you consume is packed with this toxic substance!

Also, consider the fact that cattle, sheep, chickens, etc., are naturally vegetarians. When you eat them, you are just eating polluted vegetables. Why not skip all the waste and toxins and just eat healthy, organic vegetables?

It's a myth you have to eat meat to get your protein. Farm animals, especially horses, get protein. Horses are vegetarians and get protein from grains and grasses. You can get proteins (list on next page) you need from the large variety of whole grains, soy tofu, raw nuts, seeds, beans, fruits and vegetables that God put here for us.

Meat Has Toxic Uric Acid & Cholesterol

Meat is a major source of toxic uric acid and cholesterol, both harmful to your health. **If you insist on eating meat, it should be an organically fed source and not eaten more than 1 to 2 times weekly.** Fresh fish can be the least toxic of the flesh proteins. Beware, fish from polluted waters can be loaded with mercury, lead, cadmium, DDT and other toxins. If you are unsure of the waters the fish come from, don't risk eating it.

Vegetarian Protein % Chart

LEGUMES %

Soybean Sprouts	54
Mungbean Sprouts	3
Soybean Curd (tofu)	43
Soy flour	35
Soybeans	35
Soy Sauce	33
Broad Beans	32
Lentils	29
Split Peas	28
Kidney Beans	26
Navy Beans	26
Lima Beans	26
Garbanzo Beans	23

VEGETABLES %

Spinach	49
New Zealand Spinach	47
Watercress	46
Kale	45
Broccoli	45
Brussels Sprouts	44
Turnip Greens	43
Collards	43
Cauliflower	40
Mustard Greens	39
Mushrooms	38
Chinese Cabbage	34
Parsley	34
Lettuce	34
Green Peas	30
Zucchini	28
Green Beans	26
Cucumbers	24
Dandelion Greens	24
Green Pepper	22
Artichokes	22
Cabbage	22
Celery	21
Eggplant	21
Tomatoes	18
Onions	16
Beets	15
Pumpkin	12
Potatoes	11
Yams	8
Sweet Potatoes	6

GRAINS %

Wheat Germ	31
Rye	20
Wheat, hard red	17
Wild rice	16
Buckwheat	15
Oatmeal	15
Millet	12
Barley	11
Brown Rice	8

FRUITS %

Lemons	16
Honeydew Melon	10
Cantaloupe	9
Strawberry	8
Orange	8
Blackberry	8
Cherry	8
Apricot	8
Grape	8
Watermelon	8
Tangerine	7
Papaya	6
Peach	6
Pear	5
Banana	5
Grapefruit	5
Pineapple	3
Apple	1

NUTS AND SEEDS %

Pumpkin Seeds	21
Sunflower Seeds	17
Walnuts, black	13
Sesame Seeds	13
Almonds	12
Cashews	12
Filberts	8

139

Data obtained from *Nutritive Value of American Foods in Common Units*, USDA Agriculture Handbook No. 456. Reprinted with author's permission, from *Diet for a New America* by John Robbins (Walpole, NH: Stillpoint Publishing).

Avoid shellfish – shrimp, lobster and crayfish! They are garbage-eating bottom-feeders and eat decaying scum and refuse making them an unhealthy food choice. Most poultry is commercially mass fed and heavily drugged with antibiotics and hormones. Be selective and cautious in your eating; seek only the healthiest food choices.

Don't eat pork or pork products! Pigs are the only animals besides man that develops arteriosclerosis. This animal is so loaded with cholesterol that in cold winter weather, unprotected pigs can become stiff, as though frozen solid and die. Also, pigs are often infected with a dangerous parasite which causes the disease trichinosis.

Although we feel that *meat and dairy products* are far more dangerous than they are healthy, we include this section because of this food group's prominence in the average Western diet. Meats are high in visible fat, *invisible* fat, cholesterol and toxins from the animal. That's why we stress to meat eaters not to have it more than 1 to 2 times a week and always trim off fat before cooking. Placing meat on a rack during cooking, baking or broiling helps drain off most of the fat and keeps it from soaking in its own unhealthy grease and drippings.

Don't eat greasy fried foods. The frying pan is the cradle of indigestion, heart disease and death! Those sputtering lumps of frying, sizzling fat are enemies of your heart and entire body! If you must eat meats, flavor with herbs, garlic, onions, mushrooms and Bragg Liquid Aminos, instead of fat-rich gravies. You can garnish meats with a variety of raw vegetables like watercress, parsley, celery, carrots, radishes, turnips, garlic, onions and bell peppers. Compared to meats, most fish is a better low fat protein! Buy freshly caught cold-water fish (salmon, halibut and makerel) from unpolluted waters – it's healthier.

Poultry – chicken and turkey – the organically fed and hormone and drug free are safer animal proteins. The meat is low in fat and cholesterol. Guinea hen and squab are low in fat. But duck and goose are high in fat. Discard all poultry skins and giblets because they are high in fat.

Eggs. If you do eat eggs, limit to 2 or 3 per week. Remember, yolks contain high cholesterol fat. Fertile fresh eggs from free-range organic fed chickens are best.

Chapter 13

Eat to Live – Don't Live to Eat Don't Overeat!

It's Harmful to Your Health to Overeat!

Second after second, minute after minute, hour after hour, day after day our faithful, loyal heart is working to keep us alive. In both our waking hours and during our sleep, our heart takes only a sixth of a second to rest between beats. The hardest work the heart has to do is right after an individual has eaten. The bigger the meal, the more work it has to do in pumping vast quantities of blood into the digestive tract.

Overeating puts more strain on the heart than any other one thing! Many people load up on a ten-course dinner and soon afterward suffer a heart attack! Overeating is a dangerous, deadly habit that can lead to serious consequences. You should make it a habit to always get up from the table feeling that you could eat a little more.

New studies done by the U.S. Center for Disease Control and Prevention, found that one out of five Americans are obese and the rate is climbing yearly – it's an epidemic! Obesity is defined as anyone over 30% of their ideal body weight. This leads to high triglyceride levels which can cause diabetes and cardiovascular disease.

Remember, exercise is a major key factor in lowering weight and helping keep the heart healthy and fit. Fact: only 20% of Americans exercise one hour weekly, yet they spend over 15 hours with TV and the web weekly.

Recent studies show people with large waistlines have shorter lifespans.

Sad Facts: Many people go throughout life committing partial suicide – destroying their health, heart, youth, beauty, talents, energies and creative qualities. Indeed, to learn how to be good to oneself is often more difficult than to learn how to be good to others. – Paul C. Bragg

Deep breathing is our connection to life, through the body and heart, leading us to a wholeness of being and giving us spirit for living life to its fullest. – S. Hainer

141

Current obesity studies show increases in all age groups. The biggest gain is in the 18 to 29 years old group at 12.1%, up from 7.1% back in 1991. American children (1 in 3) are more overweight than ever! The number of overweight children ages 6 to 17, has zoomed up since the 1960's. Overweight children are at high risks for adult on-set heart disease and diabetes. Teach your children healthy eating habits by being a healthy, trim, fit example for them. *(www.cdc.gov/nccdphp/dash/phactaag.htm or nutraag.htm)*

It's Proven – Light Eaters Live Longer

My father's research and interviews with people who remained vigorous at ages over 100 years revealed that they ate sparingly and never over-ate. Their diets were well balanced with simple, natural foods. Scientific tests made on controlled animal feeding have also conclusively proven that light eaters live longer and in better health.

Always *give thanks first, then eat slowly* and *chew your food thoroughly*. Never eat in a hurry! Food bolted down causes trouble and overworks the stomach and heart. Fast eating produces gas pressure on the heart and frequently heart attacks. If you don't have time to eat correctly, skip that meal! Fasting and skipping a meal is a good habit to develop.*(www.uclanews.ucla.edu/docs/ES020.html)*

Most eating habits form early in life. To live long, feel youthful and have a powerful heart you must be able to avoid and rid yourself of bad eating habits, plus condition yourself to new healthy eating habits.

A link has been found between leptin, a protein product of the obesity gene and the risk for coronary heart disease. The study was conducted by the Imperial College School of Medicine in England. The obesity gene was cloned in 1994. Its product, leptin, acts as a signal to help the body decide when it has eaten enough food to feel full. The amount of leptin in the blood has been directly linked to body fat. This study is the first to associate leptin elevations in the blood with high blood pressure. Researchers measured leptin levels in 74 men. They found that the higher the level of leptin, the more likely the risk for heart disease. Measuring leptin may become a way of determining the risk of heart disease.

Food and Product Summary

Today, many of our foods are highly processed or refined, robbing them of essential nutrients, vitamins, minerals and enzymes. Many also contain harmful, toxic and dangerous chemicals. The research findings and experience of top nutritionists, physicians and dentists have led to the discovery that devitalized foods are a major cause of poor health, illness, cancer and premature death. The enormous increase in the last 70 years of degenerative diseases such as heart disease, arthritis and dental decay substantiate this belief. Scientific research has shown that most of these afflictions can be prevented and that others, once established, can be arrested or even reversed through nutritional methods.

Enjoy Super Health with Natural Foods

1 **RAW FOODS:** Fresh, organically grown raw fruits and vegetables are always best. Enjoy nutritious variety of juices, garden salads, sprouts and raw nuts and seeds.

2 **VEGETABLE and ANIMAL PROTEINS:**
a. Legumes, lentils, brown rice, soybeans, tofu, beans.
b. Nuts and seeds, raw and unsalted.
c. Animal protein (if you must) – hormone-free meats, liver, kidney, brain, heart, poultry, seafood. Please eat these proteins sparingly or it's best to enjoy the healthier vegetarian diet. You can bake, roast, wok or broil these proteins. Eat meat no more than 1 to 2 times a week.
d. Dairy products – eggs (fertile, fresh), unprocessed hard cheese, goat's cheese and certified raw milk. We choose not to use dairy products. Try the healthier soy, nut (almond, etc.) and Rice Dream non-dairy products.

3 **FRUITS and VEGETABLES:** Organically grown is always best – grown without the use of poisonous sprays and toxic chemical fertilizers whenever possible; ask your market to stock organic produce. Steam, bake, sauté or wok veggies for as short a time as possible to retain the best nutritional content and flavor. Also enjoy fresh juices.

4 **100% WHOLE GRAIN CEREALS, BREADS and FLOURS:** They contain important B-complex vitamins, vitamin E, minerals and the important unsaturated fatty acids.

5 **COLD or EXPELLER-PRESSED VEGETABLE OILS:** Bragg Organic Extra Virgin Olive Oil, soy, sunflower, flax and sesame oils are excellent sources of healthy, essential, unsaturated fatty acids; but it's wise not to overdo oils.

143

THE MIRACLES OF APPLE CIDER VINEGAR FOR A STRONGER, LONGER, HEALTHIER LIFE

> The old adage is true:
> *"An apple a day helps keep the doctor away."*

- Helps maintain a youthful, vibrant body
- Helps fight germs and bacteria naturally
- Helps retard the onset of old age in humans, pets and farm animals
- Helps regulate calcium metabolism
- Helps keep blood the right consistency
- Helps regulate women's menstruation
- Helps normalize the urine, thus relieving the frequent urge to urinate
- Helps digestion and assimilation
- Helps relieve sore throats, laryngitis and throat tickles and cleans out toxins
- Helps sinus, asthma and flu sufferers to breathe easier and more normally
- Helps maintain healthy skin, soothes sunburn
- Helps prevent itching scalp, dry hair and baldness, and banishes dandruff
- Helps fight arthritis and removes crystals and toxins from joints, tissues and organs
- Helps control and normalize weight

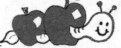

– Paul C. Bragg, Health Crusader, Originator of Health Stores

Our sincere blessings to you, **dear friends,** who make our lives so worthwhile and fulfilled by reading our teachings on natural living as our Creator laid down for us to follow. He wants us to follow the simple path of natural living. This is what we teach in our books and health crusades worldwide. Our prayers reach out to you and your loved ones for the best in health and happiness. We must follow the laws He has laid down for us, so we can reap this precious health physically, mentally, emotionally and spiritually!

With Love,

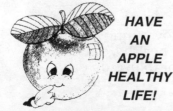

HAVE AN APPLE HEALTHY LIFE!

Braggs Organic Raw Apple Cider Vinegar with the "Mother" is the #1 food I recommend to maintain the body's vital acid – alkaline balance.
– Gabriel Cousens, M.D., Author, *Conscious Eating*

Phytochemicals - Nature's Miracles Help Prevent Cancer:

Make sure to get your daily dose of these naturally occurring, cancer-fighting biological phytochemicals that are abundant in tomatoes, onions, garlic, beans, legumes, soybeans, cabbage, cauliflower, broccoli, citrus fruits, etc. The champion – tomato, contains the highest count of miracle phytochemicals!

Class	Food Sources	Action
PHYTOESTROGENS ISOFLAVINS	Soy products, alfalfa sprouts, red clover sprouts, licorice root (not candy)	May block some cancers, & aids in menopausal symptoms
PHYTOSTEROLS	Plant oils, corn, soy, sesame, safflower, wheat, pumpkin	Blocks hormonal role in cancers, inhibits uptake of cholesterol from diet
SAPONINS	Yams, beets, beans, nuts, soybeans	May prevent cancer cells from multiplying
TERPENES	Carrots, yams, winter squash, sweet potatoes, apricots, cantaloupes	Antioxidants – protects DNA from free radical-induced damage
	Tomatoes and tomato-based products	Helps block UVA & UVB & may help protect against prostate cancers, etc.
	Citrus fruits (flavonoids)	Promotes protective enzymes; antiseptic
	Spinach, kale, beet & turnip greens	Protects eyes from macular degeneration
	Red chile peppers	Keeps carcinogens from binding to DNA
PHENOLS	Fennel, parsley, carrots, alfalfa	Prevents blood clotting & may have anticancer properties
	Citrus fruits, broccoli, cabbage, cucumbers, green peppers, tomatoes	Antioxidants – flavonoids block membrane receptor sites for certain hormones
	Grape seeds	Strong antioxidants; fights germs & bacteria, strengthens immune system, veins & capillaries
	Grapes, especially skins	Antioxidant, antimutagen; promotes detoxification. Acts as carcinogen inhibitors
	Yellow & green squash	Antihepatoxic, antitumor
SULFUR COMPOUNDS	Onions & garlic (fresh is best)	Promotes liver enzymes, inhibits cholesterol synthesis, reduces triglycerides, lowers blood pressure, improves immune response, fights infections, germs & parasites

145

HEALTHY BEVERAGES
Fresh Juices, Herb Teas & Pep Drinks

These freshly squeezed organic vegetable and fruit juices are important to The Bragg Healthy Lifestyle. It's not wise to drink beverages with your main meals, as it dilutes the digestive juices. But it's great during the day to have a glass of freshly squeezed orange, grapefruit, vegetable juice, Bragg Vinegar Drink, herb tea or try a hot cup of Bragg Liquid Aminos Broth (½ to 1 tsp Bragg Liquid Aminos in cup of hot distilled water) – these are all ideal pick-me-up beverages.

Bragg Apple Cider Vinegar Cocktail – Mix 1-2 tsp. equally of Bragg Organic ACV and (optional) raw honey or pure maple syrup in 8 oz. of distilled water. Take 1 glass upon arising, an hour before lunch and dinner.

Delicious Hot or Cold Cider Drink – Add 2 to 3 cinnamon sticks and 4 cloves to water and boil. Steep 20 minutes or more. Before serving add Bragg Vinegar and raw honey to taste. (Reuse cinnamon sticks & cloves.)

Bragg Favorite Juice Cocktail – This drink consists of all raw vegetables (please remember organic is best) which we prepare in our vegetable juicer: carrots, celery, beets, cabbage, tomatoes, watercress and parsley, etc. The great purifier, garlic we enjoy but it's optional.

Bragg Favorite Healthy "Pep" Drink – After our morning stretch and exercises we often enjoy this instead of fruit. It's also delicious and powerfully nutritious as a meal anytime: lunch, dinner or take along in thermos to work, school, sports, the gym, or to the park or hiking, etc.

146

Bragg Healthy (Smoothie) Pep Drink

Prepare the following in blender, add 1 ice cube if desired colder:
Choice of: freshly squeezed orange juice, grapefruit or tangelo; carrot and greens juice; unsweetened pineapple juice; or 1½ cups distilled water with:

½ tsp green powder (barley, etc.)	1 to 2 bananas, ripe
½ tsp raw wheat germ	1 tsp soy protein powder
½ tsp flaxseed oil (optional)	1 tsp raw sunflower seeds
½ tsp lecithin granules	1 tsp raw honey, optional
½ tsp raw oat bran	½ tsp vitamin C powder
½ tsp psyllium husk powder	½ tsp nutritional yeast flakes

⅓ cup organic silken tofu (optional)

Optional: 4 apricots (sun dried, unsulphured). Soak in jar overnight in distilled water or unsweetened pineapple juice. We soak enough to last for several days. Keep refrigerated. In summer, you can add organic fresh fruit in season: peaches, strawberries, berries, apricots, etc. instead of the banana. In winter, add apples, kiwi, oranges, pears or persimmons or try sugar-free, frozen organic fruits. Serves 1 to 2.

Patricia's Delicious Health Popcorn

Use freshly popped organic popcorn (use air popper). Try Bragg Organic Olive Oil or flax seed oil or melted salt-free butter over popcorn; now add several sprays of Bragg Liquid Aminos and Bragg Apple Cider Vinegar – it's delicious! Now, sprinkle with nutritional yeast (large) flakes. For variety try pinch of Italian or French herbs, cayenne pepper, mustard powder or fresh crushed garlic to oil mixture. Serve instead of breads!

Bragg's Lentil & Brown Rice Casserole or Soup

14 oz pkg lentils, uncooked	4 garlic cloves, chopped
4 carrots, chopped	1 ½ cups brown rice, uncooked
3 celery stalks, chopped	1 tsp Bragg Liquid Aminos
2 onions, chopped	¼ tsp Italian herbs (oregano, basil, etc.)
3 quarts distilled water	2 tsp Bragg Organic Extra Virgin Olive Oil

Wash & drain lentils and rice. Place grains in large stainless steel pot. Add water. Bring to boil, reduce heat, simmer for 30 minutes. Then add vegetables & seasonings to grains & cook on low heat until done. Just before serving, add fresh or canned tomatoes. For a delicious garnish add parsley & nutritional yeast (large) flakes. Add more water in cooking the grains to make a delicious soup or stew. Serves 4 to 6.

Bragg Raw Vegetable Health Salad

2 stalks celery, chopped	½ cup red cabbage, chopped
1 bell pepper & seeds, diced	½ cup alfalfa or sunflower sprouts
½ cucumber, chopped	2 spring onions & tops, chopped
1 carrot, grated	1 turnip, grated
1 raw beet, grated	1 avocado (ripe)
1 cup green cabbage, sliced	3 tomatoes, medium size

For variety add raw zucchini, sugar peas, mushrooms, broccoli, cauliflower. Dice avocado & tomato and serve on side as a dressing. Chop, slice or grate vegetables fine to medium for variety in size. Mix vegetables thoroughly & serve on a bed of lettuce, spinach, watercress or chopped cabbage. Serve choice of fresh squeezed lemon, orange or dressing separately. Chill salad plates before serving. Always eat salad first before serving hot dishes. Serves 3 to 5.

147

Bragg Health Salad Dressing

½ cup Bragg Apple Cider Vinegar	⅓ tsp Bragg Liquid Aminos
2 tsps raw honey	1 to 2 cloves garlic, minced

⅓ cup Bragg Organic Olive Oil, or blend with safflower, soy, sesame or flax
1 Tbsp fresh herbs, minced or pinch of Italian or French dry herbs

Blend ingredients in blender or jar. Refrigerate in covered jar.

For delicious herbal vinegar: in quart jar add ⅓ cup tightly packed, crushed fresh sweet basil, tarragon, dill, oregano, or any fresh herbs desired, combined or singly. (If *dried* herbs, use 1-2 tsps. herbs.) Now cover to top with Bragg Organic Apple Cider Vinegar and store two weeks in warm place, and then strain and refrigerate.

Honey – Celery Seed Vinaigrette

¼ tsp dry mustard	1 cup Bragg Organic Apple Cider Vinegar
¼ tsp Bragg Liquid Aminos	½ cup Bragg Organic Extra Virgin Olive Oil
¼ tsp paprika	½ small onion, minced
3 Tbsp raw honey	⅓ tsp celery seed

Blend ingredients in blender or jar. Refrigerate in covered jar.

Avoid These Processed, Refined, Harmful Foods

Once you realize the harm caused to your body by unhealthy refined, chemicalized, deficient foods, you'll want to eliminate these "killer" foods. Also avoid microwaved foods! Follow The Bragg Healthy Lifestyle to provide the basic, healthy nourishment to maintain wellness.

- Refined sugar , artificial sweeteners (aspartame) or their products such as jams, jellies, preserves, marmalades, yogurts, ice cream, sherbets, Jello, cake, candy, cookies, chewing gum, soft drinks, pies, pastries, tapioca puddings and all sugared fruit juices and fruits canned in sugar syrup. **(Health Stores have healthy, delicious replacements, so seek and buy the best and enjoy!)**

- White flour products such as white bread, wheat-white bread, enriched flours, rye bread that has white flour in it, dumplings, biscuits, buns, gravy, pasta, pancakes, waffles, soda crackers, pizza, ravioli, pies, pastries, cakes, cookies, prepared and commercial puddings and ready-mix bakery products. Also most are made with dangerous (oxy-cholesterol) powdered milk and powedered eggs. **(Health Stores have huge variety of 100% whole grain organic products, delicious breads, crackers, pastas, pizzas, desserts, etc.)**

- Salted foods, such as corn chips, potato chips, pretzels, crackers and nuts.

- Refined white rices and pearled barley. • Fast fried foods. • Indian ghee.

- Refined, sugared (also, aspartame), dry processed cereals – cornflakes etc.

- Foods that contain olestra, palm and cottonseed oil. These additives are not fit for human consumption and should be 100% avoided .

- Peanuts and peanut butter that contains hydrogenated, hardened oils and any mold that can cause allergies.

- Margarine – combines heart-deadly trans-fatty acids and saturated fats.

- Saturated fats and hydrogenated oils – enemies that clog the arteries.

- Coffee, decaffeinated coffee, China black tea and all alcoholic beverages. Also all caffeinated and sugared juice, cola and soft drinks.

- Fresh pork, pork products. • Fried, fatty, greasy meats. • Irridated foods.

- Smoked meats, such as ham, bacon, sausage and smoked fish.

- Luncheon meats, hot dogs, salami, bologna, corned beef, pastrami and packaged meats containing dangerous sodium nitrate or nitrite.

- Dried fruits containing sulphur dioxide – a toxic preservative.

- Don't eat chickens or turkeys that have been injected with hormones or fed with commercial poultry feed containing any drugs or toxins.

- Canned soups - read labels for sugar, starch, flour and preservatives.

- Foods containing benzoate of soda, salt, sugar, cream of tartar and any additives, drugs, preservatives; irradiated and genetically grown foods.

- Day-old cooked vegetables, potatoes and pre-mixed, wilted salads.

- All commercial pasteurized, filtered, distilled, white, malt and synthetic vinegars are the dead vinegars! (We use only our Bragg Organic Raw, unfiltered Apple Cider Vinegar with the "mother" as used in olden times.)

Bragg Healthy Lifestyle Eating Habits

You need to learn not only what to leave out of your diet, but also, as importantly, what you should put into it. You will find that you can nourish your body without sacrificing meal-time enjoyment once you understand the basic health principles of proper nourishment. This knowledge will show you the elements your body needs to build, develop and live healthily as it was meant to do naturally. Combinations of healthful foods packed with vital nutrients are abundant worldwide.

The first step, of course, is to get into *the habit of eating for health*. Such a habit is not difficult to form. Although the instinctive sense of food selection has been submerged with all the advertising of the popular fast, junk foods, etc. You have to be strong minded! Like any other ability or skill, a healthy lifestyle must be kept constantly in practice or its powers will deteriorate. Only by exercising this natural health instinct and desire can we revive and strengthen our health.

149

Bad Nutrition – #1 Cause of Sickness

"Diet-related diseases account for 68% of all deaths."
– Dr. C. Everett Koop

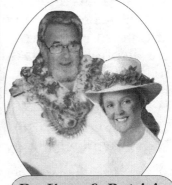

Dr. Koop & Patricia

America's former Surgeon General and our friend, said this in his famous 1988 landmark report on nutrition and health in America. People don't die of infectious conditions as such, but of malnutrition that allows the germs to get a foothold in sickly bodies. Also, bad nutrition is usually the cause of non-infectious, fatal or degenerative conditions. When the body has its full vitamin and mineral quota, including precious potassium, it's almost impossible for germs to get a foothold in a healthy, powerful bloodstream and tissues!

What a person eats becomes his own body chemistry.

Good health and good sense are two of life's greatest blessings. – P. Syrus

Proper Nutrition for Rejuvenation & Fitness

Degenerative diseases stem from breakdowns within the body, not attacks from outside, although the latter may occur secondarily as a result of weakened defenses. Since degenerative diseases arise within our bodies because of some lack of a vital element or substances, our safest course is to reinforce our defenses with those nutrients which will build our powers of resistance. *Your body is like a fortress.* Although people may look alike on the *outside, the inside* determines their strengths and weaknesses. Well-marshaled forces within a fortress can repel an enemy, while poorly organized forces will succumb. Let's build our inner strength so we will be impervious to all deadly enemies of the body!

Don't Clog Arteries with Fats & Bad Foods

As poisons accumulate in your body, it becomes impossible to have smooth, flexible arteries through which your oxygen-enriched blood can flow freely. The toxins, tars and chemicals from unhealthy foods and saturated fats and tobacco, tea, coffee and colas, leave a poisonous residue on the arteries. Not only do these fats and poisons clog your arteries, but the tobacco, coffee, tea, alcohol and cola drinks are also unhealthy stimulants to the heart. The heart has a natural rhythm which it can maintain indefinitely under most normal conditions. When you use these harsh stimulants, you actually whip and beat your heart into unnatural activity causing it to be overworked and overstressed.

Beware of "Killer" Foods

If drink can kill — so can food! Don't dig your grave with your knife and fork! To have a heart that is fit, your blood chemistry must be healthy and balanced. The 5 to 6 quarts of blood in your body must have all of the *60 nutrients that build and maintain a powerful, fit heart.*

Years ago people did not need to know what to leave out of their diet. That was because the only foods that they had to eat were those produced by Mother Nature. These foods were not robbed of their natural elements like today's foods that are processed and preserved and embalmed by the greedy food industry to stay fresh.

No One Need Suffer Heartburn

If the way to a person's heart is through their stomach, then heartburn (*acid indigestion*) is the end of the romance. Heartburn is a much misunderstood condition that has been written about since Roman times. *First*, it has little to do with the heart. *Second*, it has little to do with spicy or acidic foods. It is caused when the stomach's contents back up into the lower throat (the esophagus). These powerful stomach acids, which are stronger and more acidic than even the spiciest of foods, burn the sensitive walls lining the esophagus.

Apple Cider Vinegar Relieves Heartburn

It is vitally important that you don't join the millions of Americans who regularly take a variety of antacids, seltzers, etc. These over-the-counter medications neutralize stomach acids which only further throws off a digestive process already out of balance. You must reduce the amount of fat in your diet because fatty foods cause stomach acids to back up into the esophagus. Also, don't dilute your precious digestive juices by drinking water, juices and herbal teas with your meals. Make it a habit to enjoy beverages between (not during) meals.

When it comes to good digestion, you must practice good posture – sit up tall and straight, lifting up your chest with your shoulders slightly back. This will keep your esophagus, stomach and intestines properly aligned and will not crowd your vital machinery. Most importantly remember your stomach has no teeth! You must chew each and every mouthful of food slowly and thoroughly to a pulp (Fletcherizing) that slides down easily. This helps insure a painless, healthy digestion of your meal.

Dr. Gabriel Cousins, famous author of Conscious Eating, treats his patients heartburn with simple sips of ⅓ teaspoon of Bragg's Organic Apple Cider Vinegar before meals. Plus, do enjoy the Bragg's famous healthy delicious Vinegar Drink 3 times daily (pages 144 & 146).

Dr. Cousins says: *Bragg's Organic Apple Cider Vinegar with the 'Mother' is the #1 food I recommend to maintain the body's acid-alkaline balance which is so important!*

Olive Oil – Mediterranean's Tasty Heart Treat

Olives have been used for centuries. Not only are they eaten and used on foods and in cooking, but olive oil is used for ointments, body lotion and in many other ways. In 400 B.C. Hippocrates, the Greek physician (the father of medicine) wrote about the great curative properties of olive oil he called the *great therapeutic*. He also told of the powerful cleansing and healing properties of apple cider vinegar. (See pages 144 and 146.) *www.oliveoilsource.com*

The words of Hippocrates still hold true today. In 1994, the Lyon Diet Heart Study wanted to find out why the people of the Mediterranean region had much less heart disease than Americans and Northern Europeans. The answer was found in the characteristic diet of the region. Spanish, Italians and Greeks share a diet that is much lower in saturated fats than the diet of those regions with high rates of heart disease. The dietary fat of the Mediterranean residents is primarily olive oil.

The Lyon Diet Heart Study (For more on this study see website: www.healthwell.com/hnbreakthroughs.com/jan99/news2.cfm) and other European research has found that olive oil offers great cardiovascular rewards. After 2 years, people who decreased their fat intake and ate most of the remaining fat in the form of olive oil had a 76% decrease in new heart trouble. The greatest reduction was angina pains and non-fatal heart attacks.

Olive oil beneficially influences cardiovascular health by reducing cholesterol levels. It helps protect and strengthen the digestive system by providing the body with *polyphenols* (powerful antioxidant compounds). Don't let this delicious, healthy gift of Mother Nature pass you by! Make Bragg Organic Olive Oil a part of your diet. Dr. Julian Whitaker says it's the best for the heart.

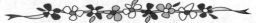

Nutritionist have been studying the Mediterranean diet for the last 20 years and have found that the residents have a very low incidence of heart disease. With the recent discovery of "good" cholesterol (HDL), scientists have begun to understand why people from the Mediterranean area have a very healthy cholesterol balance, despite their high consumption of olive oil. This is because olive oil helps stimulate body's production of "good" HDL, that helps the body limit the buildup of substances that block arteries, causing heart disease.
– Martha Rose Shulman, Mediterranean Light

Folic Acid Helps Protect the Blood

Folic acid plays a vital role in the smooth functioning of a healthy body. Long revered as a brain food, it's needed for growth of red and white blood cells and the body's energy production. Deficiencies of folic acid and also B6 and B12 can lead to serious conditions such as depression, anxiety, insomnia, immune system problems and dangerously high homocysteine levels. Two must-read books by Kilmer S. McCully, M.D. *The Homocysteine Revolution* and *The Heart Revolution* educate the reader about the deadly toxic effects of high homocysteine levels and the tragic results to the cardiovascular system.

High Homocysteine Levels Cause Heart & Osteoporosis Problems

High homocysteine levels can damage cells that line the blood vessel walls, setting the stage for future cardiovascular disease and increasing problems with diabetes, osteoporosis and kidney diseases. When having a physical, be sure to ask for a blood panel test that includes homocysteine levels. Dr. McCully says the safest and best levels are 6-8 mcm/L. Dr. White agrees (page 39).

153

For every 10% rise in homocysteine levels, there's an equal risk of developing severe coronary disease and osteoporosis. In patients with heart disease, the risk of death 4 to 5 years after diagnosis, was related to the amount of homocysteine in the plasma. Everyone produces this substance naturally, a product of protein metabolism. The homocysteine levels rise when the body is sluggish and fails to convert it to non-damaging amino acids, then they dangerously accumulate in the blood.

In most cases, therapy with various B vitamins and a healthy lifestyle menu of fresh fruits and vegetables offers the B vitamins necessary to reduce high homocysteine levels. But a "normal" American diet doesn't supply enough B vitamins to adequately detoxify homocysteine. This has been scientifically documented by Dr. McCully.

High homocysteine blood levels (safe – 6-8 mcm/L) and dietary deficiencies of vitamins (B6, B12, folic acid and CoQ10) are underlying causes of heart, osteoporosis, diabetes and kidney diseases. – Kilmer S. McCully, M.D. *(www.homocysteine.com)* and *(www.sinatramd.com)*

B Vitamins & Folic Acid Are Heart Protectors

Dr. Kilmer S. McCully pioneered the Homocycsteine Revolution and here are more positive facts: high homocysteine levels are easily corrected in most people with B-vitamins. B-6, B-12 and folic acid that helps reduce homocysteine levels in the blood. This is especially important for those who are at risk for cardiovascular problems, because 1 in every 3 people with cardiovascular disease have dangerously high levels of homocysteine. Godfrey Oakley, M.D., of the Centers for Disease Control and Prevention, says *there is strong evidence from over 200 studies that increased consumption of folic acid (from foods or supplements) will prevent cardiovascular disease.*

In addition to supplements, folic acid is found in dates, nutritional yeast, brown rice, mushrooms and more as the list shows. Folic acid works best taken with vitamin C and vitamins B6 and B12.

Some doctors prescribe short-term relief to sufferers of angina with nitroglycerin nitrolingual spray and digitalis (foxglove) medications. Both increase blood flow to the heart, but in different ways. The former relaxes the veins, increasing blood supply to the heart. The latter makes the heart muscles contract more forcefully. It's important to keep in mind that these merely offer temporary relief. The best results come from positive, healthy lifestyle changes. (see pages 207-212).

154

Healthy Food Sources of Folic Acid
— *The Health Nutrient Bible*, LYNN SONBERG

Food Source	Micrograms
Spinach, (Raw or Steamed) 1 Cup	262
Asparagus, (Raw or Steamed) 1 Cup	176
Lima beans, (Raw or Steamed) 1 Cup	156
Broccoli, (Raw or Steamed) 1 Cup	108
Wheat germ, ¼ Cup	106
Beets, (Raw or Steamed) 1 Cup	90
Cauliflower, (Raw or Steamed) 1 Cup	64
Orange (navel), (Raw or Steamed) 1 Cup	47
Cantaloupe, ½ melon	46
Cabbage, (Raw or Steamed) 1 Cup	40
Tofu, firm ½ Cup	37

Chapter 14

Doctor Fasting

Fasting – the Perfect Heart-Rester

If you are vitally interested in having a strong heart, you must skip 1 or 2 meals a week or even better, fast for one whole day out of 7. What a wonderful rest the hard-working heart receives when you take a day or 2 of total abstinence from all food! Just drink 8 to 10 glasses of cool distilled water daily. If you need something warm, have a cup of herb tea such as mint, alfalfa, anise seed, or the Bragg Vinegar Drink. You may add ½ tsp of honey to your tea if desired. During a water fast partake of no juices or food.

A Story of Successful Fasting

We have thousands of letters in our files from health students all over the world, who had remarkable recoveries with fasting. One of these students had a serious heart attack at 55 years of age. She was flat on her back in bed for 8 weeks. When she finally got up she was a pitiful sight – pale, haggard and weak. She was thoroughly discouraged since she had been told that she did not have long to live.

155

Then she got hold of our Bragg book *The Miracle of Fasting* and started to fast 1 day each week. After a few months she fasted for 3 or 4 days each month. Then she went on a 7 day fast. Great cleansing and healing took place in her body because of her fasting and living The Bragg Healthy Lifestyle. NOTE: The Bragg Book *The Miracle of Fasting* is a complete and instructive program on the Science of Fasting. See the back pages of this book for the complete Bragg book list.

Banish All of Your Fears About Fasting!

The average person has a preconceived notion that if they skip a few meals or fast for a few days, dangerous things will happen to their body. Nothing is farther from the truth! My father and I have fasted for as many as 30 days straight – and felt stronger on the 30th day than when the fast started! Caution! We don't advise our students to go on long fasts unless needed and supervised by a health professional. Inquire for good contacts at health stores, health clubs, etc. or check *www.spafinder.com*.

Nothing will give the body more energy and vitality than fasting. Fasting also strengthens the body's digestive system and heart. Forget your fears! Fasting cleanses the internal body. Try a short fast to demonstrate to yourself the miracles fasting can accomplish in your life!

Here's our personal fasting program for you: We fast on Mondays. During this time we drink 8 to 10 glasses of distilled water, 3 with Bragg Vinegar (page 146). This gives our digestive and elimination systems a complete rest. We then eat on Tuesday. This respite from food takes a great load off of the hard-working heart and digestive system and helps keep the body cleaner.

Several times yearly we take a longer *super* fast. We usually prefer a distilled water fast for 7 to 10 days. This works wonders in keeping us fit, trim and healthy (page 161)! The Hollywood Stars love juice fasting to detox (page 158).

Cleansing the Heart Pump and Pipes

If our *pipes* and great *pump* are clogged and corroded with debris and toxic poison we cannot be physically fit! Therefore, it is necessary from time to time to give the *pipes* and the *pump* of the body a thorough cleansing. This should be done by fasting once every week – for this 1 day will have beneficial effects. It will shake the toxins loose from the tissues, stimulate circulation and get rid of foreign matter that has become encrusted in the heart and blood vessels.

You should follow this cleansing program at least 1 day a week. Then in time you will have enough fortitude to fast for 3 days straight – you will be amazed at the results! If you have any reactions during this cleansing program – such as headaches, excessive gas or feeling of weakness – just remember that this is what we call a *healing crisis*. These symptoms will fade away as the toxins pass through your elimination system.

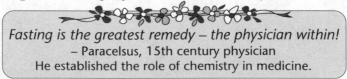

Fasting is the greatest remedy – the physician within!
– Paracelsus, 15th century physician
He established the role of chemistry in medicine.

Flushing Poisons from your Body's "Pipes"

While on this Cleansing Program, drink at least a half a gallon of distilled (purified) water daily – that is free of toxic chemicals. The night before you start this regime take 1 to 2 quarts of distilled water and add to it 2 whole carrots cut into pieces, 3 diced stalks of celery (leaves and all), 1 handful of chopped parsley and 1 beet cut up fine. *Soak this mixture overnight.* After it has soaked 10 hours or more, strain the vegetable-distilled water and discard the vegetables (great for compost). Use this water, in which the vegetables have been soaked, as part of your drinking water during first day for cleansing.

On arising have the Bragg Vinegar Cocktail (see page 146) and an hour later eat an apple and a few dried figs or dates, 1 glass of prune juice (add 1 tsp mixed oat bran and psyllium).

At 10 a.m. eat some fresh fruit (oranges, grapefruit, bananas, apples, pears, grapes) and drink a cup of herbal/green tea or *greens* drink of choice or vegetable broth. If you customarily take supplements, do so at this time.

At 12 noon have a luncheon of a tossed green salad of sliced cabbage with grated carrots and beets, chopped green onion, celery, sweet bellpepper, parsley, raw spinach, watercress, tomato and a clove of finely chopped garlic. Eat this salad with a dressing made of 1 teaspoon each of Bragg Organic Extra Virgin Olive Oil and Bragg Organic Apple Cider Vinegar or dressing on page 147. You may also have a lightly cooked vegetable (low in natural sugar) such as stringbeans, squash or any of the green leafy vegetables.

At 3 p.m. eat fresh fruit, such as apples, grapes, pears, bananas or a few dried fruits as dates, figs, prunes, etc. and a cup of hot distilled water with 1 tsp of Bragg Aminos.

At 6 p.m. have a supper of a tossed vegetable/green salad similar as lunch and a dish of lightly steamed greens (kale, mustard or turnip greens, beet tops, spinach, etc.) cooked with chopped onions, 2 cloves of garlic and 1-2 tablespoons of Bragg Organic Olive Oil. After the meal you may take your evening supplements.

Flaxseed Cleanse – optional – may take once daily:

Before dinner soak 1 tbsp flaxseed in glass of water, apple or pineapple juice. Drink or spoon eat 2 hours after meal.

Juice Fast – Introduction to Water Fast

Fasting has been rediscovered, through juice fasting, as a simple, easy means of cleansing and restoring health and vitality. To fast (abstain from food) comes from the Old English word *fasten* or *to hold firm*. It's a means to commit oneself to the task of finding inner strength through body, mind and soul cleansing. Throughout history the world's greatest philosophers and sages – including Socrates, Plato, Buddha, Gandhi and our Creator Jesus – practiced fasting and preached its benefits.

Juice bars are springing up everywhere and juice fasting has become *in* with the theatrical crowd in Hollywood, New York and London. The number of Stars who believe in the power and effectiveness of juice and water fasting is growing. A partial list includes: Steven Spielberg, Barbra Streisand, Kim Basinger, Alec Baldwin, Daryl Hannah, Christie Brinkley, Dolly Parton and Donna Karan. They say fasting helps balance their lives physically, mentally, spiritually and emotionally. Although we feel a water fast is best, an introductory liquid juice fast can offer people an ideal opportunity to give their intestinal systems a restful, cleansing relief from the high fat, high sugar, high salt and high protein fast foods too many Americans unhealthfully exist on.

Organic, raw, live fruit and vegetable juices can be purchased fresh from many Health Food Stores. You can also prepare these healthy juices yourself using a good home juicer. When juice fasting, it's best to dilute juice with ⅓ distilled water. The list on the next page gives you many combination ideas. With any vegetable and tomato combinations try adding a dash of Bragg Liquid Aminos, herbs or, on non-fast days, even some green powder (barley, chlorella, spirulina, etc.) to create a delicious, nutritious powerful health drink. When using herbs in these drinks, use 1 to 2 fresh leaves or a pinch of dried herbs. A pinch of dulse (seaweed), rich in protein, iodine and iron is delicious with vegetable juices.

Fasting is an effective and safe method of detoxifying the body – a technique used for centuries for healing. Fast regularly one day a week and help the body cleanse and heal itself to stay well. When a cold or illness is coming on, or even depression – it's best to fast! Bragg Books were my conversion to the healthy way.
– James Balch, M.D. author of *Prescription for Nutritional Healing*

Here are Some Powerful Juice Combinations:

1. Beet, celery, alfalfa sprouts
2. Cabbage, celery and apple
3. Cabbage, cucumber, celery, tomato, spinach and basil
4. Tomato, carrot and mint
5. Carrot, celery, watercress, garlic and wheatgrass
6. Grapefruit, orange and lemon
7. Beet, parsley, celery, carrot, mustard greens, garlic
8. Beet, celery, dulse and carrot
9. Cucumber, carrot and parsley
10. Watercress, cucumber, garlic

11. Asparagus, carrot, and mint
12. Carrot, celery, parsley, onion, cabbage and sweet basil
13. Carrot and coconut milk
14. Carrot, broccoli, lemon, cayenne
15. Carrot, cauliflower, rosemary
16. Apple, carrot, radish, ginger
17. Apple, pineapple and mint
18. Apple, papaya and grapes
19. Papaya, cranberries and apple
20. Leafy greens, broccoli, apple
21. Grape, cherry and apple
22. Watermelon (best alone)

Enjoy Healthy Fiber for Super Health

- KEEP BEANS HANDY, probably the best fiber sources. Cook dried beans and freeze in portions. Use canned beans for faster meals.
- EAT BERRIES, surprisingly good sources of fiber.
- INSTEAD OF ICEBERG LETTUCE, choose deep green lettuces, romaine, bib, butter, etc., spinach or cabbage for variety salads.
- LOOK FOR "100% WHOLE WHEAT" or whole grain breads. A dark color isn't proof; check labels, compare fibers, grains, etc.
- WHOLE GRAIN CEREALS. Hot, also cold granolas with sliced fruit.
- GO FOR BROWN RICE. It's better for you and so delicious.
- EAT THE SKINS of potatoes and other organic fruits and vegetables.
- LOOK FOR HEALTH CRACKERS with at least 2 grams of fiber per ounce.
- SERVE HUMMUS, made from chickpeas, instead of sour-cream dips.
- USE WHOLE WHEAT FLOUR for baking breads, muffins, pastries, pancakes, waffles and for variety try other whole grain flours.
- ADD OAT BRAN, WHEAT BRAN AND WHEATGERM to baked goods, cookies, etc.; whole grain cereals, casseroles, loafs, etc.
- SNACK ON SUN-DRIED FRUIT, such as apricots, dates, prunes, raisins, etc., which are concentrated sources of nutrients and fiber.
- INSTEAD OF DRINKING JUICE, eat the fruit: orange, grapefruit, etc.; and vegetables: tomato, carrot, etc. – UC Berkeley Wellness Letter

The best reward of a thing well done is to have done it.

Fasting Cleanses, Renews and Rejuvenates

Our bodies have a natural self-cleansing system for maintaining a healthy body and our *river of life* – our blood. It's essential that we keep our entire bodily machinery healthy and in good working condition from head to toe!

Fasting is the best detoxifying method. It's also the most effective and safest way to increase elimination of waste buildups and enhance the body's miraculous self-healing and self-repairing process that keeps you healthy.

If you prepare for a fast by eating a cleansing diet for 1 to 2 days, this can greatly facilitate the cleansing process. Fresh variety salads, fresh vegetables and fruits and their juices, as well as green drinks (alfalfa, barley, chlorophyll, chlorella, spirulina, wheatgrass, etc.) stimulate waste elimination. Live, fresh foods and juices can literally pick up dead matter from your body and carry it away. Following this pre-cleansing diet you can start your liquid fast.

Daily, even on most days during our fasts, we take 3,000 mg. of mixed Vitamin C powder (C concentrate, Acerola, Rosehips and Bioflavonoids) in liquids. This is a potent antioxidant and flushes out deadly free radicals. It also promotes collagen production for new healthy tissues. *Vitamin C is especially important if you are detoxifying from prescription drugs, alcohol or stress overload,* stated famous scientist Dr. Linus Pauling.

A moderate, well-planned distilled water fast is our favorite or a diluted fresh juice (35% distilled water) fast can help cleanse your body of excess mucus, old fecal matter, trapped cellular, non-food wastes and can help remove inorganic mineral deposits and sludge from your pipes and joints. Fasting works by self-digestion. During a fast your body intuitively will decompose and burn only the substances and tissues that are damaged, diseased or unneeded, such as abscesses, tumors, excess fat deposits, excess water and congestive wastes. (See pages 99, 175.)

Even a relatively short fast (1 to 3 days) will accelerate elimination from your liver, kidneys, lungs, bloodstream and skin. Sometimes you will experience dramatic changes (a cleansing and healing crisis) as accumulated wastes are expelled. With your first few fasts you may temporarily have headaches, fatigue, body odor, bad breath, coated tongue, mouth sores and even diarrhea as your body is cleaning house. Please be patient with your body!

After a fast your body will begin to healthfully rebalance. When you follow The Bragg Healthy Lifestyle, your weekly 24 hour fast removes toxins on a regular basis, so they don't accumulate. Your energy levels will begin to rise – physically, psychologically and mentally. Your creativity will begin to expand. You will feel like a *different person* – which you are – as you are being cleansed, purified and reborn. Fasting is an exciting and wonderful cleansing and healing miracle for your body.

BENEFITS FROM THE JOYS OF FASTING

Fasting is easier than any diet. • Fasting is the quickest way to lose weight.
Fasting is adaptable to a busy life. • Fasting gives the body a physiological rest.
Fasting is used successfully in the treatment of many physical illnesses.
Fasting can yield weight losses of up to 10 pounds or more in the first week.
Fasting lowers & normalizes cholesterol and blood pressure levels.
Fasting is a calming experience, often relieving tension and insomnia.
Fasting improves dietary habits. • Fasting increases eating pleasure.
Fasting frequently induces feelings of euphoria, a natural *high.*
Fasting is a rejuvenator, slowing the ageing process.
Fasting is an energizer, not a debilitator. • Fasting aids the elimination process.
Fasting often results in a more vigorous sex life.
Fasting can eliminate or modify smoking, drug and drinking addictions.
Fasting is a regulator, educating the body to consume food only as needed.
Fasting saves time spent marketing, preparing and eating.
Fasting rids the body of toxins, giving it an "internal shower" & cleansing.
Fasting does not deprive the body of essential nutrients.
Fasting can be used to uncover the sources of food allergies.
Fasting is used effectively in schizophrenia treatment & other mental illnesses.
Fasting under proper supervision can be tolerated easily up to four weeks.
Fasting does not accumulate appetite; hunger "pangs" disappear in 1-2 days.
Fasting is routine for the animal kingdom.
Fasting has been a common practice since the beginning of man's existence.
Fasting is a rite in all religions; the Bible alone has 74 references to it.
Fasting under proper conditions is absolutely safe.
Fasting is not starving, it's nature's cure that God has given us. – Patricia Bragg
        – Allan Cott, M.D., *Fasting As A Way Of Life*

Spiritual Bible Reasons Why We Should Fast
For a Healthier, Happier, Longer Walk With Our Creator

161

3 John 2	Deut. 11:7-15,21	Luke 9:11	Matthew 9: 9-15
Gen. 6:3	Gal. 5:13-26	Mark 2:16-20	Neh. 9:1, 20-24
I Cor. 7:5	Isaiah 58	Matthew 4:1-4	Psalms 35:13
II Cor. 6	James 5:10-20	Matthew 6:6-18	Romans 16:16-20
Deut. 8:3	John 15	Matthew 7	Zachariah 8:1

Dear HEALTH FRIEND,

This gentle reminder explains the great benefits from *The Miracle of Fasting* that you will enjoy when starting on your weekly, 24 hour, Bragg Fasting Program for Super Health! It's a precious time of body-mind-soul cleansing and renewal.

On fast days I drink 8 to 10 glasses of distilled water, some with Bragg vinegar. You may also have herbal teas and if just starting try diluted fresh juices (add ⅓ distilled water). Every day, even some fast days, add 1 tbsp. of this mixture (½ oat bran and ½ psyllium husk powder) to liquids once daily. It's an extra cleanser and helps normalize weight, cholesterol and blood pressure and helps promote healthy elimination. Fasting is the oldest, most effective healing method known to man. Fasting offers great, miraculous blessings from Mother Nature and our Creator. It begins the self-cleansing of the inner-body workings so we can promote our own self-healing.

My father and I wrote the book *The Miracle of Fasting* to share with you the health miracles it can perform in your daily life. It's all so worthwhile to do and it's an important part of The Bragg Healthy Lifestyle.

With Love, *Patricia*

Paul Bragg's work on fasting and water is one of the great contributions to Healing Wisdom and the Natural Health Movement in the world today.
– Gabriel Cousens, M.D., Author, *Conscious Eating & Spiritual Nutrition*

Take Time for 12 Things

1. Take time to **Work** –
   it is the price of success.
2. Take time to **Think** –
   it is the source of power.
3. Take time to **Play** –
   it is the secret of youth.
4. Take time to **Read** –
   it is the foundation of knowledge.
5. Take time to **Worship** –
   it is the highway of reverence and
   washes the dust of earth from our eyes.
6. Take time to **Help and Enjoy Friends** –
   it is the source of happiness.
7. Take time to **Love** –
   it is the one sacrament of life.
8. Take time to **Dream** –
   it hitches the soul to the stars.
9. Take time to **Laugh** –
   it is the singing that helps life's loads.
10. Take time for **Beauty** –
    it is everywhere in nature.
11. Take time for **Health** –
    it is the true wealth and treasure of life.
12. Take time to **Plan** –
    it is the secret of being able to have time
    for the first 11 things.

162

YOUR BIRTHRIGHT
HEALTH
CULTIVATE IT

Have an
Apple
Healthy Life!

Teach me Thy way O Lord, and Lead me in
Thy plain path. – Psalms 27:11

Chapter 15

Doctor Rest

Sound Sleep is Necessary
To Build a Strong Heart

Primitive men and women arise at daybreak and the early hours of their days are spent in vigorous physical activity. About mid-day they eat their largest meal and then immediately afterward they lie down to rest or take a nap (just as babies and young children do). In an hour or so they wake up refreshed – ready for the 2nd half of the day. Then they are active again until sundown, and shortly after sundown they go to sleep again. So primitive man is awake about 12 hours and sleeps about 12 hours.

Modern, civilized man drives himself all day under high-pressure. His day is filled with stresses, strains, worries and cares. A daily nap or *siesta* is unknown to the routine of most people. All day long he takes stimulants to keep himself going – coffee, tea, alcohol, pills, cigarettes, excessive amounts of sugar, candy, chocolate, ice-cream, etc. – everything to try to keep his poor body up to the constant *go – push mode.*

163

He lives in this hectic, fast driven age and at night he has brilliant lights and action to keep him awake. His amusements and entertainments all begin at night. The night clubs turn on bright lights and loud music. Movie theaters lure him in to films that are promoting sex, crime and violence. Television, the radio, parties – everything seems to be geared to stimulate him. Instead of going to bed for much needed sleep he drives himself, chasing happiness and peace of mind.

When he gets sleepy he just takes a pill to keep him awake or drinks some strong coffee – then to relax he has some poisonous alcohol. He is constantly straining his nervous system – all of which has a disastrous deadly effect on his circulatory system and his heart.

Think of yourself as a "battery" – you discharge energy and you must recharge yourself with proper food, sleep and constructive emotions.

The majority of American's nerves are so jangled and frazzled that it's often impossible for them to sleep. As a result, *they consume tons of sleeping pills and tranquilizers* to try to calm their exhausted nervous systems. It's no wonder that, in addition to the *soaring heart disease rate in the United States*, we have more people in mental institutions than ever before in history. A half-million American men and women are committed to mental institutions every year. These facilities are now so over-crowded that they represent one of our society's greatest medical and financial problems today. For peaceful, calm and healthy nerves read the Bragg book *Build Powerful Nerve Force*. See back pages for the book list.

Sleep is Essential To Life Itself

You cannot have a strong heart, a sound mind and a healthy nervous system if you do not get enough good and sound restful sleep! Sleep is essential to building and maintaining a strong, vital heart. *Sleep is more necessary than food!* Anyone can fast on water for days – or even weeks if necessary – without any serious harm if they are well-nourished before beginning the fast and have a satisfactory food-supply after its conclusion. But no one can *fast* from sleep for a few days without side effects. Man can't endure an entire week of sleeplessness.

In early English history condemned criminals were put to death by depriving them of sleep. Forced sleeplessness, in fact, has been used as a form of torture and execution by the Chinese and is more feared than corporal punishment. Those subjected to this always died raving maniacs! Sad facts illustrate the necessity of sleep!

Take a Daily "Siesta"

If you want to build a *strong heart* and *nervous system*, take a mid-day nap. Getting an hour's rest in the middle of the day is just like having 2 days in 1, because when you wake up after your mid-day nap or *siesta* you have stored up a terrific reserve of nervous energy. We believe the people of Mexico, South America, Spain, France and Italy had a good idea when they followed the long established policy of closing down businesses from noon to 2 pm. Rest is important for building a powerful body and heart!

How Much Sleep Do We Need?

How much sleep do we need? Every individual is different. Some people require more sleep than others. Those possessing the greatest vitality and the strongest constitutions require less sleep than those of limited vitality and weaker recuperative powers. Those who possess a strong metabolic system and great vitality can store energy during sleep and they also recover from the exertions of the preceding day more rapidly. A strong person will be restored more quickly than others. Their system can more rapidly repair the wear and tear of their daily work than that of a weaker individual.

Newest University of Chicago research has found strong signs of *accelerated* ageing in healthy young men after less than a week in which they slept for just four hours per night. Not getting enough sleep can age people prematurely and promote illness! Getting 12 hours of sleep for several nights turned the students back to their right age.

Most people need 7 to 8 hours of sleep nightly. Women and children require 9 to 10 hours sleep. We feel that 8 hours of sleep per night is important for a strong heart and that 1 to 2 hours of this sleep should be obtained before midnight. A single hour of sleep before midnight is worth 3 hours of sleep after midnight. We enjoy short afternoon naps when possible – the siesta habit is great!

165

Rules for Restful, Recharging Sleep

It's best to *sleep with your head to the north*, so you will be in direct contact with the Earth's vibrations, and on an outside porch or in a room with good cross-ventilation. Weather permitting you can sleep nude or in non-constricting natural (cotton, silk, wool) garments. Sleep with a head cradle pillow (page 166) so that your neck and spine are aligned and your heart won't have to pump so hard against gravity. Sleeping in a cramped position, on a soft mattress (firm is best) or in a manner that blocks circulation is not conducive to restful sleep. In bed, stretch and spread your body out, then practice slow deep breathing and sleep peacefully.

A study at College of Holy Cross in Massachusetts found student who got less sleep got poorer grades! Teens need 8 to 9 hours sleep per night.

Your Mattress is Your Best Sleeping Friend

You should sleep on a firm mattress or place a board under a soft one. This allows the muscles to stretch in natural relaxation and relieves pressure on vital organs.

When on our world lecture tours, we often have to move our mattresses onto the floor to be firmer. It seems that some of the world's top hotels put their money into showy lobbies and not into firm mattresses. We also often find old, sagging mattresses in many of the homes we visit – but new cars in their garages! At our Desert home we had new wood platforms made. A firm mattress goes on top of this board with four legs on castors. Try a foam *egg-crate* mattress pad on top of the mattress – it's great. It might take you a few nights to become accustomed to being stretched out flat – but soon your body will thank you with more energy.

We travel all over the world in trains, planes, ships, buses and automobiles and often use soft foam ear plugs to shut out unnecessary sounds and noises. We feel it's absolutely necessary that we sleep in a place that is quiet! Even though we often do fall asleep when there is noise all about us, the vibratory action of the noise can have a direct effect on the heart, circulation and nervous system.

We believe that individuals should sleep alone. Two people sleeping in one bed is not healthy because there are always toxins being released from the body and these toxins can be absorbed. Then there is also the noise of a person who breathes too deeply, snores (pg 168), or is restless – all of which interferes with the other person's sleep. It has been proven by scientific research that a person gets a better night's rest and stores up more vitality when they sleep alone. Married couples will wake up more refreshed sleeping next to each other – each in their own twin bed. If this is not acceptable, then a king size bed is certainly preferable to the usual small double bed.

Change your thoughts and you change your world. – Norman Vincent Peale

No one grows old by living, only by losing interest in living. – Marie Beynon Ray

Take the time to come home to yourself everyday. – Robin Casarjean

America's National "Sleep Debt"

A National Sleep Foundation poll back in 1998 discovered that a whopping 67% of American adults have a sleeping problem and that over one-third, (37%) are so sleepy during the daytime that their daily activities are interfered with. Over the past 100 years, we've reduced our average sleep time by 20% and, over the last 25 years, added an additional month to our annual work-commute time. Thus, our national *sleep debt* is rising and while our society has changed, our physical bodies and needs have not. We are paying a dear price for progress!

Getting Enough Sleep Lately?

The odds are you aren't getting sufficient sleep. American adults presently average 7 hours nightly. While everyone's sleep needs vary, scientific research indicates that we require at least 8 hours of sleep nightly.

Few are lucky enough to enjoy 5 to 6 hours of sound sleep and still perform well at work; to just get caught up, a full ten hours of rest is frequently called for!

Before Calling it a Night . . .

First make a conscious choice about how you wish to spend the 30 to 45 minutes before bedtime. Avoid a rush to *get things ready for tomorrow* or to catch up on tasks not completed during the day. Slow down your body and mind with an aroma-therapeutic/massage bath and enjoy a soothing lemon balm tea drink before bedtime and a melatonin (1mg.) cap aids sleep, plus fights free radicals.

Try Lemon Balm for a Night So Calm

Lemon Balm, whose scientific name is *melissa officianalis*, is a cooling plant with both nervine and antiseptic qualities. As a member of the Labiatae family, which also includes peppermint and spearmint, lemon balm is native to most areas of Europe and has been widely grown worldwide. Flowering between June and October, its lemon-like fragrance is unmistakable.

167

Help me to know the magic of rest, relaxation and the restoring power of sleep.

Like restful camomile, it's lemon balm's primary, volatile oils that make the plant medicinal. While appearing to be just a simple plant, it delivers a wide range of rather potent cures, ranging from stomach pain to the worst cases of insomnia. Try lemon balm tea before bedtime – miraculous results have been reported. Also, it can be blended with a variety of herbal teas. Also others to try for sound sleep are: Sleepytime, skullcap, valarian herbal teas, magnesium and calcium supplement and melatonin (1 mg) before bedtime.

Tips for Healthful Sound Sleep

- *Avoid stimulants such as caffeine, found in coffee, tea, soft drinks, chocolate, and nicotine, found in cigarettes and other tobacco products.*

- *Don't drink alcohol to "help" you sleep.*

- *Exercise regularly, be finished with your workout no sooner than 3 hours prior to bedtime.*

- *Establish a regular and relaxing bedtime routine; for example, try aromatherapy bath or shower.*

- *Associate your bed with relaxing sleep – don't use it to work or watch TV.*

- *If you often suffer from insomnia, don't take naps.*

For the Snorer in the House

Finally there is a drug-free solution (also stop all milk products and check for nose polyps) for the disturber of the quiet night, the snorer. This breakthrough is simply the nasal strip, an adhesive band-aid-like device that helps keep nasal passages open, allowing easier airflow during sleep. You can get these nasal strips in most pharmacies in sizes from small to large, depending upon the size of the snorer's nose. The cost is minimal – for just 25¢ a 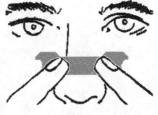 night, the snorer can often attain a more restful sleep and allow those near them to also sleep better! The snorer should stop milk (mucous forming) products and have a doctor check for nose polyps.

Chapter 16

A Frank Talk Concerning Cardiovascular Disease

Do not be discouraged if you have an ailing or damaged heart. Faithfully following our program of clean, natural living will help you to live out your entire natural life span! Yes, your miraculous body possesses tremendous recuperative powers which – if fully used – are of great help even in the most serious cases of heart trouble.

Here's Important Heart Fitness Points to Follow:

- Absolutely no smoking or drinking.
- Get plenty of sleep and relaxation.
- Don't let anybody or anything put undue pressure on you. Worry, stress, tension and strain do not necessiarily cause a heart attack – but they do not help you to avoid it either!
- Eat simple, natural, organic foods and don't overeat.

- Eat slowly and chew your food thoroughly. Chewing is first process in digestion. Saying grace helps digestion.
- Don't over-eat – it burdens your machinery and body!
- Get plenty of regular exercise. Although complete rest may be necessary just after an acute heart attack or when the heart is very weak. When this stage is past you will find regulated exercise a great help in rebuilding and revitalizing the heart and circulation.
- Don't get into emotional arguments. These waste your precious nervous energy. Walk away from unpleasant people and situations – or it's best to avoid them completely.
- Get the Happiness Habit! A cheerful, happy disposition helps promote health and longevity.
- Keep away from all artificial stimulants – coffee, china tea, cola drinks and alcohol. Do not let anyone tell you that alcohol will help your heart.
- Walk! Breathe deeply and enjoy daily brisk walks!

Healthy Heart Fitness Pointers

♥ A vegetarian diet is healthier. Instead of meat, eat unsaturated vegetarian proteins – such as soybeans, tofu, beans, raw seeds; sunflower, sesame, flaxseed, pumpkin and raw nuts such as almonds, pecans, brazil, hazel, walnut and pine nuts.

♥ Use no salt – toss salt shaker! (Use herbs/kelp/Bragg Aminos.)

♥ Eat no dairy products – milk, cheese, butter – high in clogging, saturated fats. (Use soy and rice milk products.)

♥ If you want eggs, eat only 2 or 3 a week. Organically fed free-range chicken eggs are best.

♥ Fruits and vegetables – organic, raw or lightly cooked – should form 60% to 70% of your diet.

♥ Don't use white sugar or the commercial substitutes, aspartame, etc. – they contain harmful chemicals. (Use raw honey and *stevia drops in place of sugar.)

♥ Fast for 24 hour period weekly. This gives heart and vital organs a physiological rest. It will also help reduce cholesterol and toxins in the arteries.

170 ♥ A low-fat diet, ample exercise and brisk walking with deep breathing helps you keep cholesterol levels normal.

STEVIA – World's Healthiest Sweetner

* Stevia drops (2 drops =1 tsp sugar) from a South African plant, helps regulate blood sugar and lowers blood pressure, but doesn't affect normal blood pressure. Calorie-free Stevia is suitable for diabetics, safe for children and doesn't cause cavities. It helps mental alertness, combats fatigue and improves digestion. *See www.stevia.com*

Our Opinion of Heart Transplants

When the first heart transplants were announced the newspapers reported every detail. The average person wants to hear this kind of news. They always want the easy way out. If your heart goes bad, just have another put in! Sounds wonderful! Why take care of your heart when you can get a new one when the old one falls apart? The first experiments with heart transplants were, of course, done with animals. The medical researchers reasoned that if heart transplants would work on animals, they would work on humans. Dr. Barnard of Africa performed heart transplants on 50 dogs – all died.

Heart Transplants – Risky and Costly

If success were judged during the first 24 hours after the operation, it would have been rated a success. After 2 days, complications arose, the same rejection problems that could not be solved in the animal experiments. (Interesting: pigs and human hearts are similar in size, etc.)

The body survives in a hostile environment only because it can fight off the invasion by toxic poisons, bacteria, viruses and other foreign matter. The same mechanism attacks the transplanted heart and can slowly destroy it. This difficulty was apparent also in early kidney transplants, with a survival rate of 5% (today it's 95%, but requires huge ongoing use of costly toxic drugs).

The major problem in heart and kidney transplants is tissue rejection. The body wants nothing to do with a foreign object – and that's exactly how it views the new organ! No matter how healthy the new heart or kidney may be, it's not a natural part of the body it's being placed in (Example: wood splinter in finger). To date medical science has found nothing natural – only immuno-suppressant drugs – which helps overcome this rejection of new tissues or organs by the body, and in our opinion, never will.

According to Life Magazine cover story on heart transplants, the average wait for a new heart is 207 days, which jeopardizes the waiting patient's health and results in hugh astronomical medical bills! A heart transplant operation will cost over $100,000 and to maintain it, will cost over $20,000 per year for life! Take care of your precious heart – start living The Bragg Healthy Lifestyle!

We wish that we believed these transplants will eventually work as well as your own healthy heart. (Doctos are planning to use pig hearts soon.) Today, scientific facts show that heart disease can be avoided. That's the reason our Healthy Heart Fitness Program was written, to help prevent heart conditions. We offer no cure for heart disease, only the body works the miracles!

A healthy body is a guest-chamber for the soul and a sick body is a prison. – Francis Bacon

We believe in prevention. We agree thoroughly with the American Heart Association when it says that the heart needs daily exercise and a healthy, balanced diet with ample fruits and vegetables in order to remain healthy.

Build Yourself a Healthy Heart

We do not personally believe in heart transplants. We believe that the first thing you should do is to live life so that you will not damage your heart. While outlining our Heart Fitness Program we have told you in detail about the vicious enemies of the heart. Know your enemies and keep away from them! If you have lived a haphazard life and have damaged your heart, we believe that you can still make a comeback and build a healthy heart for yourself. Remember that your body is self-cleansing, repairing and healing! Given the chance, it will do its best to rebuild a vigorous heart for you. But you must work with your body – not against it!

General public knowledge of the heart is crammed with fallacies as well as facts. Let's consider some of these misconceptions that we so frequently hear about:

Should the Heart Patient Always Rest?

No! The belief that a *coronary* always means the end of an active life is widespread – and quite wrong! Most coronary occlusions (heart attacks) involve only a small branch of the *coronary tree* or system of blood vessels. The blocked artery may be naturally bypassed by the collateral channels which lie unused in the heart tissues awaiting just this eventuality. The new circulatory route may be so efficient that the patient may have no disability at all after recovery! *Your body is a miracle.*

Certainly the process of healing is assisted if the body is rested during the acute phase of the attack. The degree and duration of any activities should be decided by your own doctor. Once healing is complete, however, further rest rarely achieves anything of value. To the contrary, it is likely to increase disability by adding the ill effects of physical unfitness and loss of self-confidence.

See your doctor if your resting heart rate is faster than 100 beats per minute.

Is Exertion Harmful After a Heart Attack?

This is a variation of the same theme as the need for rest and is usually just as wrong. The heart has enormous reserves of power which are seldom – if ever – used in ordinary living. It is this reserve which enables individuals to perform apparently superhuman feats in times of crisis or in an emergency. Athletes constantly call upon this reserve – the runner who covers a mile in 4 minutes, for example, or the 50-mile endurance swimmer.

The reserve power of the heart is not greatly decreased and is available for use even after many heart attacks. It should not be abused, of course. Generally, the heart patient who over-exerts himself will develop warning symptoms – some chest pain, angina and maybe even breathlessness. This is Mother Nature's way of telling him to slow down. Similar symptoms, however, may be the result of physical unfitness, unusual stress or tension, or emotional upsets and fatigue.

The thing we want you to remember is that *your body is always undergoing change*. You are not now the same person that you were a minute ago. The body is always undergoing endless change, for better or worse. Every moment of your life old cells are being sloughed off and new healthy ones hopefully are taking their place.

The question you must ask yourself is, *What kind of new cells am I making for my body? Am I building these new tissues with healthy food or unhealthy food?*

If you drink alcohol, coffee, tea, cola drinks and eat refined white bread, refined sugar, salted or rich, fatty foods you are going to make weak body cells that will prematurely decay, causing you health problems! On the other hand, if you follow the instructions given in our Healthy Heart Fitness Program, you are going to help build a stronger heart and a stronger body. It's all in your hands! We can only guide you to help yourself.

Stress and emotional turmoil can cause or worsen high blood pressure. Reduce stress through regular exercise, which should be a part of everyone's lifestyle for various reasons, not the least of which is lower blood pressure and improved heart health. – Health and Nutrition Breakthrough

If you have had a heart condition, start today to systematically and efficiently build a fit heart and strong circulatory system. Please don't think *a bad heart* means a permanent farewell to those healthy activities which are a major part of the enjoyment of life – it isn't!

According to studies done in the book, *8 Steps to a Healthy Heart* by Robert Kowalski, life after heart problems can be rich and fulfilling, but only if the patient and his family take the steps needed to assure that recovery includes treatment of both mind and body. Attending a cardiac rehabilitation program is beneficial for both the patient and family members, there they can share their feelings with other patients who have gone through cardiac experiences. It bridges families together and gives support to those in need. Mended Hearts, Inc. is highly recommended and offers help, support, and encouragement to heart disease patients and their families. Ask your hospital for your local Mended Hearts chapter or write them at: Mended Hearts, Inc., 7320 Greenville Avenue, Dallas, TX 75234. Or call them at 1-800-242-8721 (See *www.mendedhearts.org*)

Face the Challenge – Change Your Bad Habits

Face this challenge and start changing your bad habits of living into good, healthy habits. This is both a mental and a physical process. Your mind must control your body! Never let the body be in command! That is the duty of the mind. It must command the body to absolute obedience to its will. The whole person is at its best when mind and body work as a team. Then you can enjoy more Supreme Health!

Tell me what you eat and I will tell you what you are.
For you are what you eat! What you eat today will be
walking and talking tomorrow. – Paul C. Bragg

HEALTHY OILS RICH IN OMEGA 3 & OMEGA 6
Good for the heart & delicious on salads, greens & veggies.

	Omega 3	Omega 6
Flax Seed	57%	16%
Pumpkin	15%	42%
Soy	9%	50%
Walnut	5%	51%

Dr. John Harvey Kellogg's Famous Vegetarian Diet for Heart Patients

Dr. John Harvey Kellogg was the founder and director of the great Battle Creek Sanitarium at Battle Creek, Michigan. Sick people from all over the world – even royalty – traveled there to be under his personal care. My father was fortunate enough to work with him.

As soon as a heart attack victim was brought to the Sanitarium, Dr. Kellogg would put him on a strict vegetarian diet with the advice that this should be a lifetime diet. It was a strict, exclusively vegetarian regime consisting of fruit, vegetables, seeds and nuts. No meat, no fish, no eggs, no dairy products, no coffee, no alcohol and no salt were allowed. Dr. Kellogg believed that this strict vegetarian diet was the only one which a heart sufferer should eat because it contained absolutely no cholesterol. It was also a salt-free diet. The only drinks allowed were herb teas, fresh fruit and vegetable juices and distilled water. Dr. Kellogg told Dad that people who had come to him with serious heart damage had lived as many as 50 additional years on a strict vegetarian diet.

175

Dr. Kellogg himself lived and practiced until he was well into his 90s. He was a strict lacto-vegetarian, eating only a small amount of natural cheese and 3 eggs weekly with the otherwise completely vegetarian diet which he advocated for his heart patients. At age 92 he was still performing delicate operations at his sanitarium. Today a great many doctors and nutritionists have joined him in recommending a vegetarian diet for all heart patients.

Strokes

Every year hundreds of thousands of people become the victims of strokes. Although this disorder is frequently associated with the later years of life, this is not necessarily an affliction of old age. A few years ago, for example, a well known English motion picture actress in her late 30s had a stroke. Sadly, this has become an all too common affliction for those in their 30s and 40s.

The elimination of body toxins and waste by fasting increases longevity.
– Alexis Carrel, M.D., famous scientist

Unhealthy Lifestyles = Strokes and Heart Attacks

A stroke usually originates from the same causes as a heart attack. The arteries become clogged and narrow because of cholesterol and mineral deposits on the arterial walls, hindering the free passage of the blood. Pressure of the bloodstream trying to force its way through this blockage further irritates the walls of the arteries and creates conditions which give rise to blood clots. When a clot breaks off from the lining of the artery wall into the bloodstream it can slow or completely block the flow of blood. If a complete blockage occurs in the vital arteries that feed the heart muscle, the result is a heart attack or coronary thrombosis. If this blockage occurs in the cerebral arteries of the brain it causes a stroke, sometimes called *a heart attack in the head.*

After a stroke occurs the blood supply to a part of the brain is reduced or completely cut off. When the nerve cells in that part of the brain are deprived of an oxygenated blood supply, they cannot function and the part of the body controlled by these nerve cells cannot function either. The afflicted areas resulting from a stroke depend upon which part of the brain is affected and the seriousness or extent of the damage.

A stroke can be fatal. It can also produce paralysis of one side or a portion of the body or a single limb. A *lighter* stroke may cause difficulty in moving the arms or legs, in speaking or may result in a loss of memory.

After the stroke, the damaged nerve cells may recover or their functions may be taken over by other brain cells. Some victims may suffer such serious damage that it will take a dedicated effort to make even a partial recovery. It's important that immediate attention to proper diet and exercise begins! We have seen miracles with stroke victims regaining full use of affected muscles. Physical therapy and massage treatment should be begun soon as possible to aid rehabilitation and speed recovery! Prolonged inactivity impairs the circulation and makes recovery more difficult. The victim can use his own hands (even if one hand) to massage affected areas 4 to 6 times daily and help bring them back to health.

Bright's Disease – Dropsy, Swollen Legs & Ankles

When the small arteries of the kidneys are affected by this same blockage problem it produces a condition known as *dropsy* or Bright's disease. The most noticeable symptoms are swelling of the legs and ankles. Although this painful swelling (called *edema*) does not always indicate Bright's disease, this ailment is so widespread and insidious that it must be suspected and a physician consulted immediately. Whether the thickening and blockage process takes place in the heart, head or kidneys, it's essentially the same disease. It is refered to as atherosclerosis by doctors. This means that the arteries that carry the blood are blocked with the hard, waxy trouble maker – cholesterol.

See web: *www.drchristopher.com/ailments/BRIGHTS_DISEASD.html*

Prevention is Far Better than Cure!

. . . and generally more successful! That is why we keep stressing your living The Bragg Healthy Lifestyle! You must banish from your head the notion that age alone damages your heart and blood vessels. Remember that age is not toxic. It's not a force, but a measure. Live so well that you will never suffer a stroke or a heart attack! You now know what your enemies are – tobacco, excess weight, stimulants such as coffee, tea, alcohol and cola drinks, fatty – unhealthy foods, sugars, table salt and salty foods and lack of daily exercise. Take heed and action!

Pacemakers Save Lives When Needed

Famous Doctor Earl Bakken pioneered the first transistorized pacemaker. Medtronic, the company he co-founded, has further developed the pacemaker for ailing hearts that has and is saving thousands of lives. Doctor Bakken and his lovely wife live in Kamuela, Hawaii where he is pioneering a holistic hospital that integrates natural healing therapies to bring the patient back to health. They are Bragg Olive Oil, Apple Cider Vinegar and Bragg Amino users. (www.fivemtn.org/fivemtn/people/bakken.html)

Stress puts an unhealthy strain on the heart. A UCLA study found 6 out of 10 heart patients had constricted arteries and reduced blood flow to their heart following any emotionally charged upsets or events.

Sponging the body with cold water and apple cider vinegar is an excellent skin tonic for helping with dropsy and Bright's Disease. – Dr. John Christopher

Follow This Heart Fitness Program

This Heart Fitness Program is designed to help you build a stronger heart and a more youthful circulatory system. Mother Nature cannot be pushed or rushed – but if you will cooperate with her, you can have *the heart of a lion*. If you have a weak heart or weak *pipes* that are clogged, remember that it took a long time to get them into that condition. You must be patient with Mother Nature while the regeneration, rejuvenation and cleansing processes take place within your body.

A fit, youthful heart can be yours, if you are willing to work for it! No one else can make your heart strong. It depends entirely on you. Your eating habits, lifestyle and your physical activity will determine the type of heart and health you will enjoy.

Enjoy Positive Thinking and Positive Action

To have a healthy and powerful heart you must develop strong willpower. You must overcome all negative thoughts about the *inevitable* impacts that age supposedly ravages on the heart and body. Do not let cowards and weaklings influence you away from following this Healthy Heart Fitness Program! These fear mongers will try to impart their fear to you by telling you to go easy on exercise, fasting and life changes. Don't believe them! Have faith in your ability to improve!

When following this Heart Fitness Program and lifestyle you are working with Science and Mother Nature. Don't let unqualified people influence or deter you! Years of research and investigation have gone into the development of this Heart Fitness Program in order to provide you with a master plan for building a strong, fit heart for a long, fulfilled, healthy life.

Prevention is always preferable to the cure.

To our minds the greatest mistake a person can make is to remain ignorant when he is surrounded, every day of his life, by the knowledge he needs to grow and be healthy, happy and successful. It's all there. We need only to observe, read, learn and apply. – Paul C. Bragg

Men do not die, they kill themselves. – Seneca, Roman Philosopher

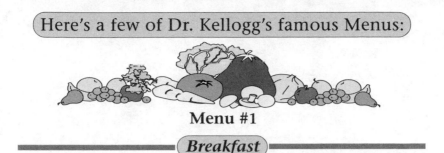

Menu #1

Breakfast

Natural Sun-Dried Apricots* topped with
Raw Wheat Germ and
Sliced Banana or Orange (if desired)
(*soak in jar overnight in distilled water or
unsweetened pineapple juice)

OR

you may substitute any morning the
Bragg Health Pep Drink on page 146
for a delicious energy breakfast. Remember to
first earn your breakfast with some exercise.

Lunch

Bragg Raw Vegetable Combination Salad
Grated Raw Beet, Carrot, Cabbage, Zucchini,
Chopped Tomato, Green Onions and
Sprouts: Alfalfa, Mung or Sunflower

Healthy Salad Dressing
made of Fresh Lemon or Orange and Bragg Olive Oil
(Also try Flaxseed or Hempseed oil)
with a dab of raw Honey

¼ Cup of Raw Sunflower or Pumpkin Seeds
(rich in Protein and Natural Oil)

Raw Apple

Dinner

Tossed Green-Leaf Salad
with Raw Spinach, Kale, Cucumber, Celery,
Parsley and Tomato

Protein – Tofu or Cooked Rice with Beans or Lentils

Fresh Fruit

Here's more of Dr. Kellogg's famous Menus:

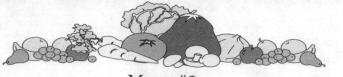

Menu #2

Breakfast

Apple Sauce*
Steel Cut Oats– hot cereal**
served with Honey, Blackstrap Molasses,
Pure Maple Syrup or Stevia (page 170)
100% Whole Wheat or Rye Toast
(*Make your own Apple Sauce, if desired add Honey)
(**Top and serve with Sliced Ripe Banana or other Fruit)

Lunch

Bragg Raw Vegetable Combination Salad
(Same as 1st Day)
Vegetable Soup with Natural Barley and Lentils
Whole Rye Toast or Oat Bran-Raisin Muffin

Dinner

Cabbage, Apple & Carrot Cole Slaw with Spring Onions
Brown Rice or Baked Potato with Skin
Baked or Steamed Carrots and Peas
Fresh Fruit
OR
Avocado, Red Onion and Tomato Salad
Steamed Asparagus or Broccoli
Raw Nuts of any kind
Fresh Fruit

"There is but one way to live and that is Mother Nature's and God's Healthy Way!"

Nutrition directly affects growth, development, reproduction, well-being and the physical and mental condition of the individual. Health depends upon nutrition more than on any other single factor. – Dr. William H. Sebrell, Jr.

Studies show both beta-carotene and vitamin C, abundantly found in fruits and vegetables, play vital roles in preventing heart disease and cancers.

Potassium Helps Strengthen the Heart

Take an extra ½ tsp of apple cider vinegar in ½ glass distilled water, twice daily between meals – good before exercise. But also enjoy your basic 3 vinegar cocktails daily (pg 146).

The heart is a large muscle and your master pump. It uses large amounts of potassium to keep going strong and healthy, hour after hour, for your entire life! It is the hardest working muscle in the body. The heart must have a constant, continuous supply of power and energy to continue beating. Apple cider vinegar contains natural potassuim that combines with healthy heart foods to make the heart muscle stronger and also help to normalize blood pressure and cholesterol.

Potassium is the Master Mineral

Potassium is an essential mineral for the body because it puts toxic poisons in solution so they can be flushed out of the body. **The body is self-cleansing, self-correcting, self-repairing and self-healing!** Just give it the tools to work with and you will have a painless, tireless, ageless body, regardless of age! Forget calendar years, for age is not toxic! You age prematurely when you suffer from potassium deficiencies and malnutrition. This low Vital Force and waste buildup (poor elimination) allows disease to proliferate.*

The Bragg Healthy Lifestyle will help you rebuild your Vital Force. Watch the transformation that will take place in your body when you faithfully follow your ACV regime. You can, and will create the kind of person you want to be! It's exciting to plan, plot and follow through!

Although you must follow this program closely, do not try to do everything listed here immediately. Remember, it took you a long time of living by wrong habits to cause any of the problems your body might have now. So, it's going to take time for the body to cleanse, repair and rebuild itself into a more *perfect health home* for you! Please remember, your body is your temple while on this earth – so cherish it and protect it!

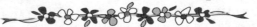

* See the website: www.healthcentral.com/mhc/top/002413.cfm#Definition:

Six Points to a Healthy Heart

We bring you this book not so much to help you as to help you help yourself. If we repeat certain points, it is with the zeal with which one taps a nail already driven home. Our main objective is to inspire you to a more intense enthusiasm for living The Bragg Healthy Lifestyle and health and to warn you against certain dangers which you may easily overlook. Throughout this book we have tried to strongly stress these 6 points:

1 You have but one heart and one life – you should take care of these priceless treasures!

2 Your body must obey the commands of your mind, for flesh is dumb and needs a health captain!

3 Every bad habit that weakens your heart and shortens your life must be broken and then banished forever!

4 You should demand of yourself a higher living standard for more health, peace of mind and happiness!

5 You should regard your body as you would a fine instrument or precision machine whose care and control is in your capable hands!

6 You must draw closer to Mother Nature and God so as to keep your life simple as 1,2,3 as your years increase!

Let us, then, throw ourselves into Their loving and understanding arms! Try to understand and follow Their wise laws and live as They wants us to live – in superb health for a long, active life of helping this world to be a better, safer, healthier place for us all.

The Complete Naturalist

The complete naturalist's goal is to identify so completely with Mother Nature that self and world become one. To do this, keep your life simple as 1, 2, 3, filled with peace, joy and love. Then with serene, clear-eyed confidence put yourself into Mother Nature's and God's hands to run your machine, heal your hurts and comfort you in sickness and adversity. When your time and usefulness on Earth is ended, you'll be called home for eternity in heaven. Psalm 23 is soothing and positive.

Let your body be nourished by natural food, pure distilled (rain) water, fresh air and gentle sunlight. Exercise and relax your body and let Mother Nature do the rest! Treat your body with the same care and wisdom that you would a champion animal. Surely as your animal will take prizes, so will you! It is easy to sneer at *health-minded, back-to-nature* people. We who believe in God and Mother Nature will enjoy long, happy, healthy lives.

Get Close to Mother Earth and God

It is good to establish contact with Mother Earth, her soil, water, air and sun. Let your bare feet grip into the soft grass and to feel soft mud or sand and squish it between your toes! We love gentle sun (before 10 a.m. or after 3 p.m.) and air baths with few clothes on. We love exercising, stretching, walking and swimming on the beach beside a sea, lake or river. Keep in close touch with Mother Earth and God, letting Their strength and virtue pass into you through your skin and bare feet! *Modern living can complicate our lives with hot house living conditions!* Man was a healthier, happier creature when he lived simpler and closer to Mother Nature.

Just stand on any big city street and watch the people rushing past. You will see that 3 out of 4 of them are probably sick, fat or physically unfit. Very rarely do you see a super healthy specimen! Don't be like the average sick or half-sick person. They have never known the real thrill of healthy living! Most people today are addicted to some kind of chemical substance such as tobacco, coffee, tea, alcohol, cola drinks and even some drugs. People turn to drugs when their vitality hits bottom. When health is gone, vitality goes with it and the zest for living. These lost souls turn to drugs in an effort to get false *thrills and kicks* out of life.

CoQ10 Combats Heart Disease, Cancer, Gum Disease and Ageing:

Dr. Stephen T. Sinatra's CoQ10 recommendations:
- 90-120 mg daily as preventive in cardiovascular or periodontal disease
- 120 to 240 mg daily for angina pectoris, high blood pressure, cardiac arrhythmia and gingival gum disease
- 240 to 450 mg daily for congestive heart failure and dilated cardiomyopathy

– Dr. Stephen T. Sinatra, author, *CoQ10 Phenomenon* www.sinatramd.com

Follow the Laws of Mother Nature and God

In the past it was the middle-aged and older people who felt they had to seek drugs or other artificial means to hang onto life. Now, tragically, young people are using drugs of all kinds. They are throwing away their natural vitality and turning their backs on Mother Nature. Now youths have become candidates for heart attacks. The heart is damaged by these stimulants and depressants.

The further we get away from living according to The Laws of Mother Nature and God, the sicker we get physically, mentally, emotionally and spiritually.

One of the dominant themes of this book is the idea that building a powerful heart at any age is a gradual return to a more natural form of living. Use natural healthy foods, vigorous exercise, deep breathing, restful sleeping, loose clothing and beautiful simplicity of life to reach a closeness to Mother Nature and God that makes you almost one with Them! You will never have a weak, sick heart if you live close and in partnership with Them. When you can feel the same strong, pure, elemental forces that manifest themselves in a pine tree expressing themselves in you, then you are on your way to positive, strong health principles.

Begin to live as Mother Nature and God want you to live. Try to feel that They claim you and that you are part of all the glad and growing things on this Good Earth! Put yourself into Mother Nature's and God's hands. We are all eager to aid you on the path to Supreme Health!

It's Up To You To Be Happier and Healthier!

Actions speak louder than words and can elevate your mood if you feel depressed. Take a walk and do slow, deep breathing – it helps you sort out and solve problems. Spend time with children – it simplifies life and puts everything in perspective. Find the comics in the newspaper or something funny to read and laugh about. If someone is upset, try to analyze the situation from that person's perspective. Make yourself physically smile and laugh; it opens blood vessels in the back of your head to physically lift your mood. Choose to be happy in spite of circumstances. No one "makes" you happy – it's an attitude you self-create from within. – Paul C. Bragg

Open your eyes so you may behold wondrous things out of thy law. – Psalm 119:18

Time flies, but remember you are your human vehicle's navigator.

Chapter 17

The Art of Longevity

The best recipe for a long life is to keep living The Bragg Healthy Lifestyle. There is no substitute for this!

Consider each day a little life in itself – make it as perfect and well-rounded as you can! Try to have a stronger heart and better health on your next birthday than you have today. By living supremely for the moment you are living superbly for a long, healthy, happy future!

You must always be self-aware of your life! The moment you relax your guard the enemy is ready to rush in and smite you in your heart. True, with luck, you may live long without trying, but you will live longer and better if you exert an effort. Living for longevity is an art. The person who deliberately sets out to prolong their days has a healthy chance of doing just that!

Forgetfulness of self may make the time go like magic, but it does not help build a strong heart and keep you youthful. Inattention to yourself and the carelessness that results is extremely dangerous! As you live longer you should grow less objective and more subjective. The more self-centered you are, the better you will conserve your precious health resources. Longevity often belongs not to those who forget themselves for others, but to those who are most health conscious of themselves and their physical, mental, spiritual and emotional well-being.

This may seem to give the long-lived a positive, strong, at times selfish character. Not at all! Without healthy nourishment we cannot aspire to fulfill our dreams. To seek to prolong one's life is to extend one's term of usefulness and service. We aren't advocating you prolong your life at the expense of others! Rather, we suggest that you live a long, healthy life so that you may be more useful to others, as well as to yourself!

185

It's important for people to know what you stand for. It's equally important that they know what you won't stand for. – Mary Waldrip

May your years be 120. – Genesis 6:3

Do You Show Signs of PREMATURE AGEING?

Is everything you do a big effort?

•

Have you started to lose your skin tone?
Muscle tone?

•

Do small things irritate you?
Are you forgetful? Confused?

•

Have voices begun to fade?

•

Has your vision started to dim?

•

Do you wobble a little when you walk?

•

Do you get out of breath
when you climb stairs?

•

How limber is your back?

•

Do your joints creak?

•

How well do you adjust to cold and heat?

•

Ask yourself this important question:
Do I seem to be slipping and
not quite like myself anymore?
If the answer to this question is "Yes,"
You had better do something about it!

START TODAY
Living The
Bragg Healthy
Lifestyle!

LOSS OF TEETH • THINNING • HAIR OF • FADING OF SIGHT • SALIVARY GLANDS SHRINK • LOSS OF HEARING • HIGH BLOOD PRESSURE • STIFFENING OF JOINTS

186

Dear friend, I wish above all things that thou may prosper and be in health even as the soul prospers. – 3 John 2

Secret of Longevity – Organized Resistance

The secret of longevity is to understand that *the enemy is not your chronological age. Premature ageing is preventable!* You must put up a strong defense against ageing. There are a few, of course, who are born with such wonderful constitutions `they simply can't kill themselves. You might find a few octogenarians who say they owe their long life to smoking, alcohol and avoiding exercise. You can tell them confidently that they could extend their lifespan by a good 20 years by living a healthy lifestyle.

Scientific longevity is organized resistance. It is based on a knowledge of the body and the laws of health. Above all, it means reliance on Mother Nature. She abhors ill health, which is another name for toxic poisoning and clogged pipes. She is always striving to purify and to vitalize. She wants to help you if you will only let her. Medicine, drugs and doctors will do you no good if Mother Nature is not backing them up.

Heart Disease is Your Greatest Threat

Remember that you must always defend yourself against coronary thrombosis (heart attack), stroke, hypertension (high blood pressure), arteriosclerosis (hardening of arteries), atherosclerosis (blockage and clogging of the arteries by cholesterol and other debris), angina pectoris, varicose veins and other cardio-vascular (heart and blood vessel) diseases. *Diseases of the heart and circulatory system are the #1 Killer in the United States* taking more than a million American lives each year – more than all other causes combined! And never forget that you must also guard against stiffening joints, fibrous tissues, deafness, blindness and many other enemies of health and life.

All this means that there must be a little slowing of activity. We believe the advice *grow old gracefully* is wrong! Mother Nature and God will eventually decree the end – but until then it's far better to live life as youthfully as possible ! You are *as old as you feel – so feel young!* When you abide by Mother Nature's Laws, you feel younger! By trusting in and obeying Her laws, understanding your miracle physical machine and how to care for it, you can live a long, youthful, healthy, happy life.

Old Age is Not Inevitable – Scientists Say Man Should Live to 140 to 185

It seems to us that what we call *old age* is the result of sluggish cell action in the body. The cells are being renewed all the time by the moisture in the lymph circulation, just as a tree is renewed all the time by the circulation of its sap. But if the cell is clogged in any way by toxic deposits which it cannot be completely rid of – chiefly because of poor circulation of the blood – it cannot then make full use of the building material brought by the lymphatic system or the nourishment and oxygen delivered by the bloodstream.

On the basis of what we have done with rabbits, we have come to the conclusion that if we can do the same thing for man, he can live a healthy and normal life until the age 185! A waxy material, cholesterol, is deposited on the arteries and there is a correlation between age and the amount of cholesterol deposited. In tests of 52 rabbits, we have been able to reverse the symptoms of old age! says a brilliant Brooklyn Polytechnic Institute Biochemistry Professor, Dr. W. M. Malisoff, who did extensive research there.

Biologists tell us that man grows an entirely new body every 11 months. That being the case, why does mankind age? Scientists answer this by saying that the body fails to shed all of the old cells. As we stated earlier, deposits in the cell prevent its full use of the new material. So instead of living 7 times the period it takes him to mature, as most animals do, man's life is unnaturally shortened by his unhealthy lifestyle. Sad facts!

Confirmation of this statement comes from Dr. Serge Veronoff of Paris, France, who says that each of us should live to be 140 years old. A human being matures at 20 years of age. Mother Nature constructed the human machine to live 7 times that age, or 140 years. The fact that some men and women even today have been able to reach or surpass the age of 120 years and have then died of some disease seems to prove the validity of the 140 year life-span without disease as natural.

#1 Cause of Death – Coronary Disease

Deposits in the arteries retard the circulation of the blood. The speed and efficiency of the bloodstream has a great effect upon the prolongation of life. It is the bloodstream which provides the entire body with the required nourishment and oxygen before it removes harmful substances for elimination. Slowing of blood circulation, loss of elasticity of blood vessels and disturbances of the machinery which regulate distribution of blood are among the most important causes of the shortening of life, vigor and health.

In our opinion, there is no physiological principle limiting health or human lifespan. We believe that radiant health and youthfulness is within reach, but it must be earned. This is your life! It is your sacred duty to yourself, Mother Nature and God to learn now and how to keep your body healthy and fit for a long lifetime.

The #1 cause of widows and widowers in the United States is coronary (heart) disease. Remember our discourse of cholesterol, and the fact that high cholesterol levels are invitations to heart attacks? Statistics show that cholesterol levels in American men, and now women also, increase rapidly between ages 30 and 65. Be on guard! Cholesterol should be tested by all twice a year.

Women before the age of 50 used to be much better protected against degenerative artery disease than men. Today women have almost achieved an unfortunate equality by developing heart attacks and strokes with nearly the same frequency as men. The scientific theory that female sex hormones play an important part in providing protection against the harmful menace of atherosclerosis is apparently true – but not powerful enough to offset the deadly effects of an unhealthy lifestyle! As soon as menopause starts in women, the protection of these sex hormones ceases, they claim, and they become just as susceptible as men to heart attacks and strokes. It's important, women of all ages should not neglect their heart health. (I've never taken hormones – only supplements and occasionally use wild yam cream – page 213.)

189

Unhealthy Lifestyle Living is Slow Suicide

Just because you are *feeling fine* does not mean that you can afford the risk of continuing to choke your bloodstream with the high cholesterol diet typical of most people in our *modern* civilization. Bacon and eggs, meat and potatoes, pies and cakes, bread with butter or margarine, milk and ice cream, all the rich foods that most men and women crave are slow poisons to your heart and circulatory system. Remember that these poisons work silently and insidiously. Their effect may not become evident until you suddenly have a heart attack. Always remember the words of Dr. Paul D. White:

– that death from a heart attack is not sudden it's been building up for years!

Your Family's Life is in Your Hands

We would like to suggest to everyone that you re-read Dr. White's warning and that you take it seriously. If you want to keep your family alive, work on them to exercise every day as you watch what you feed them and yourself. You may be shortening the lives of your family with too many fattening and highly saturated foods. Their lives are in your hands! You prepare and put the food on the table for your family to eat. You will learn from this valuable book how to keep your family in perfect health. Follow these instructions and soon you and your family will discover a startling increase in vigor and vitality, with a sense of well-being.

Remember that young people can also die of heart disease! Teach your children how to eat correctly. Give your family more fresh salads, more lightly steamed vegetables, more fresh fruit desserts. Eliminate the gravy (it's loaded with cholesterol). Eliminate dairy products. Enjoy healthier soy, rice and nut milks. Serve delicious herbal teas such as mint, alfalfa, chamomile, lemon balm, anise seed and banish coffee and the salt shaker from your table. Your reward will be a radiantly happy, healthy family. Use Bragg's *Health Gourmet Recipe Book* or the *100% Vegetarian Recipe Book* healthy ways to feed yourself and family! (See back pages for book list.)

Enjoy Lighter, Smaller Vegetarian Dinners

It seems to be an American custom for people to eat their biggest meal in the evening. From a standpoint of heart attacks, this is the worst time to eat a big meal . . . especially a meal with a preponderance of fat. It has been definitively established by researchers that the blood is more likely to clot 2 to 8 hours following a meal with a high fat intake. It would therefore seem logical to avoid heavy meals – particularly in the evening – to minimize the chances of intravascular clotting. The occurrence of a heart attack after eating a heavy meal has been recognized by doctors for years. Just think how often you read or hear about a man in his prime dying of a heart attack during his sleep at night.

Retired people, of course, can regulate their mealtimes easily. Business people can dine at an earlier hour in the evening and can certainly regulate their diet to promote their health and prolong their lives.

A light healthy vegetarian meal is ideal for evenings.

191

It can begin with a raw combination salad with lemon and olive oil dressing. Follow it with 2 lightly cooked vegetables such as stringbeans, zucchini, peas, corn on the cob, kale, okra, vegetable chop suey, etc. Several nights a week add a baked potato – but do not drench this potato in fat! Season it with a spray of Bragg Aminos, sea kelp and Bragg Organic Olive Oil instead of butter.

Now we are not telling you that the price you must pay to avoid a heart attack and live a longer life is to give up good flavor. Not at all! As mentioned previously, delicious French dishes, soups, salads, potatoes, veggies, etc. are world famous and among the best heart-healthy recipes. A good French chef rarely uses salt and cooks with very little fat. The secrets of French flavor lie in the use of herbs, garlic, olive oil, onions, green peppers and mushrooms.

I've seen sickness and asthma disappear completely in response to major shifts in diet and lifestyles, such as eliminating sugar and meat and switching to a healthier, vegetarian diet. – Dr. Andrew Weil, www.drweilselfhealing.com

Prevention is always preferable to the cure!

Chinese Recipes Promote Heart Health – America's Coronary Disease Rate is Ten Times Higher than China!

The Chinese have a low cholesterol, low fat diet – in sharp contrast to the high cholesterol, high fat diet found in the United States, Canada and the more prosperous countries of Europe. Pathologists, scientists and medical researchers have produced overwhelming evidence that when blood cholesterol and fats are high, the arteries suffer from a greater degree of atherosclerosis. *Atherosclerosis has always been a "disease of the rich".* Only those who could afford rich, fatty foods have been heart attack and stroke victims. The heart and blood vessel degenerative diseases have historically been associated with royalty and wealth. Cholesterol was found in the mummies arteries of the Pharaohs of Egypt, whose diet was far richer than their subjects.

Today we have millions of people in our Western industrialized countries who can easily afford rich foods. You hear and read about *the affluent society and its blessings.* But this affluence is exacting a high price in atherosclerosis and the nearly epidemic number of heart attacks, strokes and cancers now happening worldwide.

Millions of people living in China and other Asian countries are rarely afflicted with heart disease. Their main dietary item is, and has been for centuries, one of the most healthful of all vegetables: the soybean. Soybeans contain a high percentage of unsaturated fatty acids and lecithin, two good preventors of heart disease.

The basic Chinese diet consists of rice and lightly cooked vegetables, with meat used only as an occasional flavoring. When you order chicken or beef chop suey in a Chinese restaurant, you always get a plentiful dish of vegetables such as celery, onions, green bellpeppers, bamboo shoots, water chestnuts and soy and bean sprouts – flavored by only a very small amount of finely sliced chicken or beef and a dish of rice. No bread and butter is served at an authentic Chinese Restaurant.

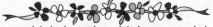

You are what you eat, drink, breathe, think, say and do. – Patricia Bragg

Our Favorite Chinese Recipes
Raw Combination Garden Salad

Slice cabbage into bite-size pieces. Add sliced carrots, celery (greener the better), turnips, radishes, cucumbers, tomatoes, fresh chopped parsley and spinach. Toss with a dressing of Bragg Liquid Aminos, Bragg Organic Olive Oil and Bragg Apple Cider Vinegar or fresh lemon juice.

Mushroom Chop Suey

With a sharp knife slice onions, green bell peppers, celery, chard or kale, carrots, bok choy, cabbage and any other vegetables you desire. Mix with fresh or canned bean sprouts, water chestnuts, bamboo shoots. Try a variety of fresh mushrooms. Put these mixed vegetables into a hot wok or skillet with a small amount of unsaturated oil such as olive, corn, soy or safflower oil. Fresh sliced garlic may be added if you enjoy it. (We do. We feel that garlic purifies the body's pipes and helps boost your immune system.) Stir in 1 teaspoon of Bragg Liquid Aminos or spray it over the chop suey just before serving for a delicious natural seasoning flavor.

The secret of Chinese food is not to overcook it. Sauté this chop suey mixture 8 to 12 minutes at the very most, stirring constantly with a wooden spoon.

Healthy Organic Brown Rice

Brown rice is a healthy staple food. Use natural organic brown rice – 1 cup of rice to 3 cups distilled water. Add ½ teaspoon Bragg Liquid Aminos and 1 teaspoon Bragg Organic (extra virgin) Olive Oil. Cook in a double boiler or in a thick-bottomed pan with tight lid, over medium heat until rice is soft and fluffy (30 minutes). Don't stir until ready to serve, then add another dash or spray of Bragg Liquid Aminos and a sprinkle of Brewer's Yeast (large flakes) for a delicious flavor. Serves 3 to 4.

Fresh Fruit Dessert

A fresh organic apple, pear, banana or any other fresh fruit in season will top off this perfect heart-smart meal.

You Can Teach Old Dogs New Tricks

They say you *can't teach an old dog new tricks*. We feel wise, mature humans have the intelligence to protect themselves from heart attacks by learning new tricks of eating. It's worth the effort to know that you are not going to wake up one night gasping for air and clutching your heart! Start now improving your daily lifestyle habits!

To avoid heart attacks you must learn to substitute Bragg Organic Olive Oil instead of butter, margarine and other clogging, saturated and hydrogenated fats. If you are a milk drinker, learn to substitute the rice, almond or soy milks and drink these instead of cow's milk. Learn to use herbs, kelp, garlic, onions, Bragg Liquid Aminos and other natural ingredients to add delicious flavors and aromas instead of salting your foods. Also, you know the saturated fats in meats, eggs and dairy products are your enemies! Learn to eat them sparingly or not at all! *Keep your meals as natural and simple as possible.*

Most people shake their heads in doubt when they are told they must give up using salt. It does take a little time to make the change from salt to naturally delicious and nourishing herbs, kelp and Bragg Aminos. We told you that the salt craving is acquired and not natural. It will disappear, just as Dad's cravings did. You will find that your 260 taste buds will soon reject salted foods.

Stop Heart Trouble Before It Starts

It's your life, the one you have until heaven calls. It's your heart and you only get one good one. Remember, when you satisfy an unnatural appetite for health-destroying foods, you are actually helping to destroy your best and most essential vital organ – your own heart! We believe it is far better to make a few changes in your diet than to drag around a paralyzed arm, leg or body as a result of a stroke, or to have your life cut short by a heart attack! So stop this very minute for a meditation period and have a heart to heart talk with yourself! Make up your mind that you're not going to die from a heart attack or be crippled by a stroke!

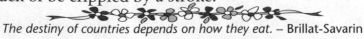

The destiny of countries depends on how they eat. – Brillat-Savarin

Feel Youthful Regardless of Your Years

Life is the survival of the fittest and no one – yes, no one – is going to be able to protect your heart except you! It's your duty and responsibility to yourself to live a healthy lifestyle so that your heart can remain strong and healthy throughout your entire natural lifespan.

We must live by knowledge and wisdom – not by old wives' tales and myths. That is why this book was written: to provide the scientific facts about your heart and outline a Heart Fitness Program that helps you take care of this marvelous, life-giving machine.

This book's message is simple. It tells what a heart attack is, what causes it and what you can start doing today to prevent it. We offer no magic formula or cure for heart trouble. In this Heart Fitness Program we have simply brought together well-documented evidence from the great scientific and medical researchers, statisticians and dietitians of the world. The medical world is relying upon heart transplants and drugs. We are not the least interested in heart transplants nor are we interested in the diagnosis and treatment of heart troubles. We are mainly interested in disease prevention by keeping the heart healthy and fit. Let's stop heart troubles before they start! Why wait for the heart to deteriorate before we do something about it? We must live well today so that we do not have a heart attack tomorrow! What we sow in one period of our lives we reap in another. Let's sow the seeds of good health so that we will automatically have a powerful, fit heart.

You can definitely capture and retain the joyous feeling of youthfulness no matter what your calendar years may be! By living The Bragg Healthy Lifestyle outlined in this Heart Fitness Program, you can again feel the joy of youthfulness and boundless energy.

Don't let people drag you down to their low level of thinking. *You are as young as your arteries!* Decide that you are going to live a healthful life to help keep your arteries and heart years younger. Keep your *thinking* youthful and you will feel young again! Age is not birthdays – it's a matter of how well you live, feel and enjoy each day of your life!

195

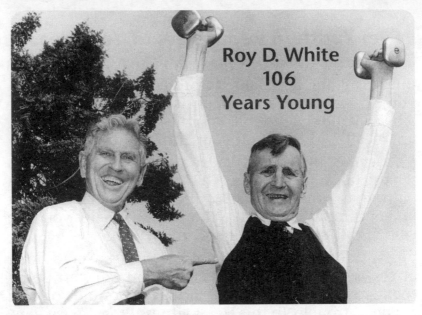

Roy D. White
106
Years Young

Paul C. Bragg With His Youthful Friend

Roy just celebrated his 106th birthday – yes, you read correctly – 106 years young! Roy D. White lives in Long Beach, California. He has a keen brain, a great sense of humor and a feeling of youthfulness tingling throughout his supple, straight and active body. Roy can lift both hands high overhead, keep his knees stiff and bend over and touch his toes – an exercise people half his age cannot do. And he never fails to walk his 5 miles a day. Being a widower, Roy takes care of his own apartment and prepares all his own meals. At 106, he appears to be a youthful, active 75 years young and even with the physical agility of a man many years younger.

Remember that throughout this Heart Fitness Program we have stressed how important it is to keep physically active. Our claims are backed up by this 106 year old youngster! Don't let your circulation slow down.

To over-rest is to rust and rust can lead to destruction.

Roy believes his daily brisk walks help him physically, mentally, emotionally and spiritually. He believes you can walk off your tensions and worries. Roy says, *I've always been free from tensions – that's the foundation of my Philosophy of Life. Fear and hatred are the two worst things in the world. You can multiply your troubles by thinking they're worse than they are – no matter how mean anyone has been to me, I've never hated them. Let them do the hating, not me!*

Tensions, anger, greed and excessive emotionalism can damage your heart! Roy is an example of the great philosophy of forgiving and forgetting. He says that most young children think that way and he wants to always be kind and think youthful. When you have such a strong sense of well-being and optimism, your entire attitude toward life is fresher and more youthful. Your whole philosophy can change to a younger and more optimistic one, replacing the stagnating defeatist attitude that so many people have. When you feel youthful, you act youthful and above all you think to live youthful!

It's Never too Late to Think Youthfully

The whole Heart Fitness Program is designed to make you forget birthdays and live a more youthful, carefree life. Living by this philosophy of life prevents many physical and mental miseries that are likely to afflict older people. In this way you can maintain health, strength, vigor and happiness as the years roll by. It has been said that *There is really no cure for old age – only those who die young escape it*. But our Heart Fitness Program can really help you feel younger and live longer.

197

We No Longer Celebrate Birthdays

That is absolutely right. No more birthdays for us! We no longer want to measure our lives by calendar years – only biological years.

Yes, we both have lived wonderful long lives. Dad to a great-great-grandfather. But this does not stop us from enjoying our youthful activities. We're going to continue to play tennis with the youngsters, climb the mountains with the mountain climbers, swim with the swimmers and dance with our young health friends – and the seniors who are still young at heart! One of Dad's favorite dancing partners is a girl of only 88 – but what a dancer! She is as graceful as any of his great granddaughters!

Don't think the years are making you old – it's the way you live that preserves or damages your heart and arteries. You must earn your bonus years! You must earn your youthful arteries! You must work hard to preserve the vitality and the fitness of your heart and body!

It's wonderful when you build up a fit heart and body, for then you find more time and energy for so many more activities than you did when you were stumbling around tired and only half-alive. When you have a heart that is beating joyfully, the world looks like the Garden of Eden. You become a carefree person with a song in your heart, a sparkle in your eye and a spring in your step. Life can be beautiful – for when you're healthy, you're happy! After all, is that not the greatest goal in life – *sweet, contented happiness and inner peace!*

Now Get Started – For Life is Precious

Start this very minute on your Heart Fitness Program! Get it firmly in your mind that you're going to build a fit heart! Banish all negative thoughts! Have faith . . . for you are now going to work with a powerful force – Mother Nature and God. Say to yourself day after day, *I am building a healthy, strong, fit heart.* Think strength and vitality for your heart.

You must be the *Captain of Your Health* at all times. You are surely more powerful than any cup of coffee, more forceful than tobacco, alcohol, salt, fat and other toxins that help to destroy your health and heart! Take command of your body and mind today and let nothing distract you from following your Heart Fitness Program!

If you feel yourself weakening in your resolve, look to a Higher Power for courage and willpower. You were given one heart, one body, one life by your Creator . . . and you were given Mother Nature as your ally to help you achieve a long, healthy and happy life. But no one – not even God or Mother Nature – can make you help yourself. You must do it – now get started!

> **Ten Little, Two-Letter Words of Action To Say Daily:**
> ## If it is to be, it is up to me!

No man can violate Nature's Laws and escape her penalties. – Julian Johnson

Professor A.E. Crews of Edinburgh University, who studied both worms and animals, stated: "Given appropriate and essential conditions of the environment, including proper care of the body . . . Eternal Youth can be a reality in living forms! It's been found to be possible, by fasting, to keep a worm alive 20 times longer than normal. This has also been proven with animals." See web: *www.walford.com* for more on this subject.

Chapter 18

Chelation Therapy

Miraculous Method of Unclogging the Arteries

We want to share with you a miracle of medical science which we found so amazing that we researched it thoroughly. We have found mounting impressive clinical medical evidence, by our personal investigation, demonstrating a safe and reliable therapeutic method to counteract the terrible ravages of arteriosclerosis and atherosclerosis. These degenerative diseases arise from hardening and clogging of the arteries.

This method is Chelation (pronounced key-lay-shun) Therapy. It has been proven effective to the point of being termed *miraculous* by physicians as well as patients. *It's totally incredible!* declared John, the first chelation therapy patient we interviewed. We met John through a mutual friend from Chicago, who was visiting us at our desert home in California. He insisted that we go to John's home in nearby Palm Desert to learn firsthand of his friends *miracle cure* and it was a miracle for sure!

199

A leading heart specialist had told John, a man in his 40s, that he had a life expectancy of maybe 2 years unless he underwent drastic surgery for a *3-way bypass;* i.e., transplanting blood vessels from his leg into his heart to bridge or *by-pass* blockages in 3 arteries (with 100%, 95% and 75% blockages respectfully). Even if he survived the surgery, there was no guarantee that similar blockages would not re-occur, leaving John in despair.

Through friends he learned about Ray Evers, M.D., who for many years had been achieving remarkable recoveries in similar cases with chelation therapy. The average treatment period is 3 to 8 weeks and can be handled on an out-patient treatment at any of the doctors' offices or clinics that perform chelation therapy.

We met John 3 months after he had an 8 week series of chelation treatments under Dr. Evers' care. He had just had a checkup at Loma Linda Hospital and the tests showed no heart or circulatory problems whatsoever!

Reversal of the "Ageing Process"

Shortly thereafter, we visited with Dr. Ray Evers at his Meadowbrook Hospital in Belle Chasse, Louisiana. He told us that over a period of 8 years he had treated over 10,000 patients with chelation therapy. Dr. Evers said that he believed *Chelation therapy could hold the key to the basic treatment of some of mankind's greatest killer diseases, all characterized by the same basic abnormality – that is, narrowing and closing off of the blood vessels, which can affect the health of every organ of the body.*

Everyone is familiar with the clinical picture of coronary or heart attacks, strokes or brain clots and hemorrhages, he continued, *but many other diseases such as diabetes, thyroid and adrenal disturbances, digestive problems, Alzheimers, senility, emphysema, arthritis, multiple sclerosis, etc., may also be caused, at least in part, by interference with the proper delivery of blood to the needed vital structures.*

Chelation therapy attacks this basic problem of the cardiovascular system, Dr. Evers pointed out. *The results often produce significant relief of symptoms, are often life-saving and sometimes miraculous.*

We saw proof of his words with our own eyes. We observed people in their 40s to their 80s being brought into the hospital in wheelchairs – the victims of heart attacks and other circulatory or degenerative diseases such as stroke, diabetic gangrene, crippling arthritis and senility. Several weeks later we watched these same people walking out of the hospital with a new, reborn spring in their step, aglow with the joy of living.

Beware of Deadly Aspartame Sugar Substitutes!

Although its name sounds "tame," this deadly neurotoxin is anything but! Aspartame is an artificial sweetener (over 200 times sweeter than sugar) made by the Monsanto Corporation and marketed as "Nutrasweet," "Equal," "Spoonful," and countless other trade names. Although aspartame is added to over 9,000 food products, it is not fit for human consumption! This toxic poison changes into formaldehyde in the body and has been linked to migraines, seizures, vision loss and symptoms relating to lupus, Parkinson's Disease, Multiple Sclerosis and other health destroying conditions (even Gulf War Syndrome). Learn more information about this crime against our health. For more info on this killer check these websites: www.aspartamekills.com, holisticmed.com/aspartame and bragg.com

What Causes This Amazing Rejuvenation?

The arteries of these people were being unclogged by chelation therapy, cleansed of the accumulated debris that had hardened and thickened the walls of these vital blood vessels. Now that their *pipes* were opened wide, the blood could once more course through their arteries, veins and capillaries to bring life-giving oxygen and nourishment to every cell in their body and carry off toxic wastes. The process of degeneration . . . commonly called the *ageing process* . . . was being reversed!

What Mainly Causes "Ageing?"

As we discussed earlier in this book, the so-called *ageing process* is not the result of the passage of time, it is primarily the result of inadequate blood circulation, which can and does occur at any calendar age. *The chief villains are an excess of inorganic minerals, calcium, etc. and toxic chemicals (of which undistilled drinking water is a primary source), combined with an excess of cholesterol from a diet rich in saturated animal fats and hydrogenated fats and living an unhealthy lifestyle.* All add to *ageing process*.

Arteriosclerosis, or hardening of the arteries, results from calcium deposits on the arterial walls. With the onset of deadly atherosclerosis, the calcified walls are further thickened by waxy deposits of cholesterol, dangerously narrowing the passageway of the blood.

The calcium seems to act as a cementing agent, forming plaques with the cholesterol, to which other inorganic minerals and waxy fats attach themselves. The narrowing of the lumen, or passageway, lessens both the quantity and force of the blood flow. Body cells degenerate from lack of nourishment and drown in their own toxins, causing many of them to die.

Vitamins, minerals and superfoods optimize your healing potential. They offer potent armor to deal with the body-ageing realities of today's environment: mineral depleted soil, strong toxic chemical use, oxygen robbing pollutants, etc. Fortifying your diet with supplements and superfoods strengthens your health and ability to function in a world which makes it tough to be healthy.
– Linda Page, N.D., Ph.D., Author of *Healthy Healing* • *1(888) 447-2939*
See Doctor Page's interesting website: www.healthyhealing.com

---

Studies show low CoQ10 levels cause heart disease, periodental conditions, declining memory and brain function. CoQ10 helped reverse these conditions.
–Dr. Stephen T. Sinatra, author, *CoQ10 Phenomenon* www.sinatramd.com

Chelation – Safe, Effective & Inexpensive Treatment For Coronary Heart Disease

Chelation therapy is a therapeutic adaptation of a natural biochemical process. The term *chelation* derives from the Greek word *chele* (pronounced keely) meaning a crab-like, pulling claw. Without going into detailed chemistry, chelation in human metabolism is the process by which an enzyme grabs or *blinds* an organic mineral or *metal* and transports it to the body part where it can be utilized or removed. Example: Zinc to the pancreas for making insulin; and iron for the hemoglobin (red blood cells); calcium for building bones and its many other body uses; etc. (Remember, this refers to organic minerals – not inorganic, which cannot be used.)

This natural chelation process was not discovered until the 1940s. Its first therapeutic application was during World War II after a synthetic chelating agent was created to act as an antidote for *mustard gas* and other forms of arsenic poisoning. (For 20 years thereafter, chelation (pulling) agents were developed almost exclusively for ridding the body of toxic heavy metals such as lead.)

In late 1950 they discovered chelating agents used as poison antidotes were also effective in removing inorganic calcium deposits from the body's joints, organs and cardiovascular system. Through studies and medical research, a safe, effective chelating agent, known as EDTA by Abbott, was produced for removing these inorganic calcium clogging deposits and cholesterol plaques from the arteries and flushing them out the kidneys.

EDTA, a natural amino acid chelating agent, does not affect the normal organic calcium utilized by the body, but chelates only pathological inorganic calcium deposits. Chelation has proven an effective way to reverse hardening of the arteries. It unclogs the arteries by chelating out these atherosclerotic plaques, which then dissolve and break up. The cholesterol and other deposits then become slushy and are easily flushed out. All the residue *goes down the drain* and then the *pipes* of your cardiovascular system become free flowing.

Life is a song, love is the music.

Chelation Therapy Includes a Healthy Diet

Carlos P. Lamar, M.D., of Florida, pioneered chelation therapy since 1960 and developed the basic procedures which have been so successful to date. These include the proper dosage of Endrate (ETDA) – delivered slowly intravenously, lasting from 3 to 4 hours per treatment.

As an essential part of chelation treatment, Dr. Lamar and his colleagues prescribe an anti-atherogenic diet that naturally chelates. Patients eat more frequent, lighter meals (with more tropical fruits; bananas, kiwis, mangos, papayas and pineapples, rich in the enzyme bromelain that acts like cardiovascular pipe cleaners) and eliminate dairy foods and saturated fats. Emphasis is placed on fresh, organic fruits and vegetables and natural foods.

Also, 50 to 100 mg supplement of vitamin B6 (pyridoxine) is mandatory (controls sodium/potassium blood levels, helps produce red blood cells and hemoglobin and protects against infection), plus additional vitamin and mineral supplements for each patient when needed.

Safe Diagnosis with Non-Invasive Tests

All patients are given thorough physicals and tests before the start of chelation therapy, and are carefully monitored during the chelation treatments, and given complete instruction for follow-up procedures. We were impressed with the infrared thermographic scan, which is diagnostic equipment that provides a safe, accurate method of locating and determining the degree of arterial blockage. Formerly this was done only by the dangerous angiogram test. This scan is a heat-sensitive instrument which records body temperature with direct correlation to blood circulation. This thermogram reveals location and degree of blockage by a light spectrum with a 10-color range. We don't recommended taking the risk of an angiogram. We endorse the non-invasive tests and the infrared thermographic scan on pages 35 to 38.

We must always change, renew, rejuvenate; otherwise, we harden. – Goethe

Bragg Books can be your faithful health guides, by your side night and day.

Chelation Therapy Promotes Natural Healing

Because it attacks the basic cardiovascular problem of degeneration, chelation therapy helps regenerate the body's natural self-healing and repairing powers. Natural blood circulation restores normal metabolism and biochemical functions. The whole body *comes alive.* This is why chelation therapy, from the very beginning, has exceeded the wildest expectations of medical science.

When the first cases were reported in 1964 by Dr. Lamar in the national medical publication *Angiology* (Vol. 15, No. 9, September 1964), the most surprising result was the significant decrease in the insulin requirement of diabetics in response to chelation therapy. Two of the early cases were *hopeless* elderly diabetics with extreme mental deterioration and severe cardiovascular complications. After treatment there was a complete remission of symptoms, both physical and mental – plus a marked decrease in their insulin requirement. This *bonus* was attributed to the increased circulation in the pancreas, which promoted insulin production.

Since then, chelation therapy has been found to achieve such *bonus benefits* as regeneration and rehardening of bones weakened by osteoporosis, restoration of mobility to frozen osteoarthritic joints, relief from hypothyroidism, reversal of prostatic calcinosis, recovery of normal functions of the kidney, other glands and organs and improvement in deteriorated retinas. There was improvement in all pathological conditions resulting from impaired circulation!

Chelation (ETDA) treatment has proven to be effective in treating heart disease. It also has achieved marked improvement in patients suffering from 2 of the most baffling central nervous system diseases – multiple sclerosis and Parkinson's disease. Perhaps the most spectacular results of chelation therapy are evidenced by the restored mental acuity in advanced senility cases.

In a landmark study, Dr. Carlos Lamar stated in the *Journal of the American Geriatric Society* (Vol. XIV, No. 3, 1966), *"The physical rehabilitation and enjoyment of living experienced by these patients would be impossible to match through any other available therapeutic procedure."*

A Universal Need for Chelation Therapy

As early as 1968, Dr. Lamar predicted, *"I have little doubt that eventually new ligands (chelating agents) will be created that will be effective by the oral (natural supplements) route. That will be the big step that will bring chelation therapy to the reach of any patient suffering from any form of calcific disease, plaque and cholesterol build-up."*

"The great advance in preventive medicine lies in clearing the arteries of deposits which close them BEFORE the symptoms or attack which make the disorder obvious to everybody," Dr. Evers declared. *"This is where chelation therapy has its greatest future."*

There are hundreds of chelation clinics in America and around the world. The best web source of doctors for chelation therapy is ACAM (the American College for Advancement in Medicine), 23121 Verdugo Drive, # 204, Laguna Hills, CA 92653. USA (800) 532-3688 and for CA and Foreign (949) 583-7666. For list of doctor members see web: *www.acam.org* where you can see the doctors in your area by zip code, also doctors around the world.

205

In Europe, world famous Dr. Claus Martin has the vision, wisdom and education to direct his *In Four Seasons Clinic* in the Bavarian Alps where he provides chelation, oxygen and life cell therapy. These are remarkable life-prolonging treatments that help reverse age-related and degenerative cardiovascular diseases. Hollywood Stars, Famous Statesmen and other noteworthy people have and are reaping the benefits of his treatments. He is a long time highly respected member of ACAM. There are over 200 chelation clinics throughout Europe. Checkout the ACAM website or if in Europe write or call:

Dr. Claus Martin, M.D.
Box 244, D-8022 Rottach-Egern, Germany 83700;
FAX 011-49-80-222-4740; PHONE 011-49-80-222-6780.

Harvard cardiologist Herbert Benson conducted experiments with thirty hypertensive people who knew nothing about meditating. After he taught them how, he discovered that their blood pressure did indeed go down. The blood pressure of those people who continued daily meditating and praying went down to normal. If they stopped the practice, it began to rise again.

Healthy Heart Facts

Dr. Roy Walford, a famous Life-Extension Researcher at University of California, Los Angeles is a leading Scientist in dietary-restriction studies who practices it himself and never overeats. He was the head scientist of the Biosphere Study in Arizona. This experiment involved 4 men and 4 women living in a totally enclosed environment for one year. Their calories were restricted by 29%. During that time they all registered healthier, decreased levels in blood pressure, triglycerides, cholesterol and other toxins! www.walford.com

Thirty years ago most medical schools taught that any cholestrol reading below 350 mg/dl was acceptable. The consensus today is that the level should be much lower – below 200 mg/dl for adults.

Researchers have discovered that the more healthy habits an individual practices, the longer they live and the healthier they are!
– Elizabeth Vierck, *Health Smart*

When you have been stricken by illness, your new car, your new home, your new big, bank balance – all these fade into unimportance until you have regained your vigor and zest for living again. – Peter J. Steincrohn, M.D.

The heart that loves is always young. – Greek proverb

*Love doesn't make the world go round.
Love is what makes the ride worthwhile.* – F. P. Jones

The Bragg Healthy Lifestyle followed daily will help you enjoy a long healthy life!

A man is as old as his arteries. – Virchow

We know two things about how to prevent death in middle age: smoking and cholesterol. – Richard Peto, Oxford University

The nation badly needs to go on a healthy diet. It should do something drastic about excessive, unattractive, life-threatening fat. It should get rid of it in the quickest, safest possible way and this is by fasting. – Allan Cott, M.D.

Difficulties strengthen the mind as labor does the body.

Medicine is only palliative. For behind disease lies the cause, and this cause no drug can reach. – Dr. Weir Mitchell

The digestive organs of coffee drinkers are in a state of chronic derangement which reacts on the brain, producing fretful moods. – Dr. Bock, 1910

Enter – or perhaps re-enter – the brave new world of wellness through exercise, natural remedies, alternative therapies, meditation and positive thinking.
– Monica Skrypczak

Chapter 19

Herbs – Garlic – Food Supplements Mother Nature's Healers

Our book gives you a program for healthy and rewarding living. When you follow The Bragg Healthy Lifestyle you can build a strong and healthy heart. This takes you down the path to increased confidence, creativity and vitality! Please remember, you can always strive to live a more healthy, positive life.

In building a healthier and stronger heart don't forget the miraculous healing gifts available from Mother Nature's kingdom. For thousands of years people around the world have used herbs and plants as medicines, tonics and remedies. Many of them are renowned for increasing heart health. Today, scientific research supports the traditional use of many of these medicinal plants. Herbs such as garlic, ginko, hawthorn, bilberry, gotu kola and rosemary have been traditionally used and scientifically researched for the treatment of heart and circulatory conditions. Here's a brief description of some of the most effective herbs. In addition to The Bragg Healthy Lifestyle, make use of these miracles of the plant world for your heart's health and fitness. Remember to consult your health care professional before substituting herbs in a previously existing condition. The key to a healthy heart is prevention and The Bragg Healthy Heart Program.

207

Garlic – The Herb that Lowers Cholesterol

Garlic is one of nature's great miracles. No other medicinal plant is more effective in the treatment and prevention of atherosclerosis! No wonder there has been increased research involving garlic and cardiovascular health. Research shows eating garlic regularly decreases serum cholesterol and dangerous triglyceride levels! People who eat garlic regularly have healthier arteries and blood than those who don't. This is why people in France, Greece, Italy, etc. (who traditionally eat lots of garlic) have a lower incidence of heart attack and disease than people in the United States.

Garlic – Your Body's Health Friend

Back in 1993 an extensive revealing study on garlic in the *Annals of Internal Medicine* found that even small amounts of fresh garlic eaten daily can significantly lower cholesterol levels in people with high cholesterol levels. Other exciting studies show that garlic helps decrease the blood's bad LDL-cholesterol levels while increasing levels of good HDL-cholesterol! It's also a general blood tonic. Garlic can lower your high blood pressure, inhibit blood clotting and improve your blood flow by reducing your blood's viscosity. Please make garlic part of your daily routine for better heart health! We use fresh garlic! *http://www.balchmd.com/link1.cfm?ART_ID=4*

Ginkgo – Improves Blood Flow to Brain

Over the last 40 years, Ginkgo has been one of the most scientifically researched medicinal herbs in the world today. Scientists know that *Gingko Biloba* (leaf) *Extracts* (GBE) dilate arteries, capillaries and veins, which increases blood flow. Therefore GBE reduces blood clotting and clogging of the arteries. GBE's strong cardiovascular benefits are localized in the brain. Increasing evidence supports the GBE effectiveness in treating ailments associated with too little blood flow to the brain (such as short-term memory loss, senility, short attention span and depression). Look for GBE supplements in health stores. *http://www.ginko-biloba.net/extract.html*

Hawthorn – Great For Preventing Angina

As we said before, angina pectoris results when one of the heart's arteries is temporarily deprived of oxygen. The artery goes into a spasm that causes a sharp pain in the chest. Angina is recognized as a warning signal and a common precursor of heart attacks too. The Hawthorn Berry is used in Europe and China for heart and circulatory ailments. Also use as a preventative as part of a healthy heart lifestyle. Scientific studies show hawthorn's ability to dilate blood vessels (especially coronary vessels associated with angina). It also helps to strengthen the heart and normalize the blood pressure.

Cayenne Promotes Healthy Circulation

People worldwide use a variety of hot peppers in their cooking. Peppers are also firmly rooted in traditions of folk medicine. When we talk of cayenne pepper, we are referring to a number of red hot peppers of the genus, *capsicum annuum* – which includes cayenne, the famous Tabasco pepper, Mexican chili peppers, pimiento, the Louisiana long pepper and others. All contain *capsaicin,* the pungent substance that gives hot pepper its kick and the most important of its medically active ingredients.

Prior to the Civil War the red pepper had gained a reputation in the U.S. as a heat rub when applied to the skin. Since then people have found that it promotes health and healing in many ways! Example: cayenne has become popular as a digestive aid and a pain reliever salve for injuries, arthritis, etc. For arthritis, osteoarthritis, joint pain and stiffness, try glucosamine and chondroitin sulfates and MSM combo. These help heal, regenerate and soothe. Also try capsaicin and DMSO lotions (pat lightly).

Cayenne is a powerful heart and health healer, so make use of it's potential! Studies confirm cayenne's effect as a general blood tonic, linking it to a reduction of blood clotting. These studies show capsaicin (cayenne) has beneficial effects on the cardiovascular system, lowers cholesterol levels and helps prevent heart disease. (See page 16) For healthy heart benefits add cayenne flakes to food regularly to season: soups, potatoes, vegetables, salads, beans, rice, etc. instead of salt! Or take cayenne supplements. Try this; 1 tsp. Bragg Aminos, ½ lemon, tiny pinch of cayenne flakes in a cup with hot water.

www.healthyideas.com/healing/herb/971118.herb.html

What Are Free Radicals?

Today there's much talk about free radicals – the toxic oxygen molecules that attack the body's cells. These dangerous substances (page 210) cause health problems and early ageing. The health risk they pose is so great that Dr. Julian Whitaker, editor a health newsletter says,

Free radicals are the primary cause of heart disease – the #1 health problem facing the world today! – Dr. Julian Whitaker

Life-Saving Antioxidants are Life-Savers

Antioxidants are compounds that prevent free radicals from damaging your body! Both antioxidants and free radicals are naturally produced by your body. You can tip the scales in your favor by increasing the vital antioxidants in your body through a diet rich in vitamin C and E, barley grass, beta-carotene (found in green leafy vegetables, yams, sweet potatoes, carrots, etc.), and flavonoids (found in grapeseed extract, bee pollen, propolis, milk thistle, ginkgo, etc.). The danger of free radicals is immense, so please maximize your intake of antioxidants (through good nutrition and supplements*****) and minimize your exposure to toxic free radical catalysts.

Free Radical Catalysts Are Deadly

These substances are dangerous sources of free radical contamination. Exposure to them exacerbates the dangers that free radicals (#1 cause of ageing) pose to your health. It's absolutely essential you eliminate (or limit!) your exposure to these toxic free radicals:

- **Aluminum** – antacids, deodorants, baking powder, tap water, deodorants, cans, foils, pots and pans, and in many drugs
- **Cadmium** – batteries, cigarette smoke, coffee, gasoline, and metal pipes
- **Carbon Monoxide** – auto exhaust, cigarette smoke, smog
- **Chlorine** – tap water, swimming pools and table salt
- **Copper** – tap water, toothpastes and dental work
- **Lead** – dyes, gasoline fumes, paint, plumbing, auto exhaust
- **Mercury** – amalgam (silver) fillings, fish, paint, cosmetics
- **Nitrates and Nitrites** – used in many processed foods, meats, etc. as a preservative. Also found in tap water.
- **Petroleum Products** – fuels, solvents, polishes, paints, and pesticides
- **Polynuclear Hydrocarbons** – fried, deep-fried and char-broiled and barbecued foods
- **Radiation** – environmental radiation, radon, televisions, and cellular phones
- **Synthetic Drugs** – antibiotics, painkillers, barbiturates, and in a host of other products

*__*__ SOD, super oxide dismutase, is an antioxident that neutralizes the free radical so that it is no longer a danger to the body. **Vitamin A** protects mucous membranes from damage, helps improve night vision, makes gums and tooth enamel stronger and has many overall health benefits.*

B-Vitamins Important for Healthy Heart

Evidence shows certain B-vitamins help reduce the risk of heart disease by lowering the harmful amino acid *homocysteine* from the blood (It's not in Bragg Aminos). Too much homocysteine brings damage to cells lining blood vessel walls. Harvard study shows B vitamins (B1, B3 *niacin*, B5 *pantothenic acid* , B6, B12 and folic acid) reduce homocysteine. See pages 153-154. *www.homocysteine.com*

Plant foods are major sources of vitamin B6 and folic acid. However, vitamin B12 is not found in vegetables. Vegetarians can obtain sufficient B12 from tofu and other soybean products; or from vitamin supplements. We recommend brewer's yeast (also known as nutritional yeast), a delicious flavor enhancer rich in B-vitamins (except for B12). Nutritional yeast is great for pets too! (Helps keep fleas away.) In the Bragg household we sprinkle delicious nutritional yeast (large flake variety) over salads, soups, veggies, potatoes, tofu, rice, beans, etc. and popcorn. See our delicious popcorn recipe on page 146.

211

Vitamin C is for Capillaries and Cholesterol

For your capillary/health, turn to vitamin C. Thousands of studies conclude vitamin C makes healthier capillaries by reducing clotting in the bloodstream. Remember, your blood must move along your capillaries in single file, cell by cell. A blood clot can completely stop the flow of blood through these microscopic vessels! Researchers recently attributed other cardiovascular benefits to C, including clearing of cholesterol and calcium from arterial walls. It's a strong weapon against hardening and clogging of your arteries. Taken before bedtime, studies show it prevents heart attacks during sleep and in the morning. This new info supports studies conducted 40 years ago by pioneering Doctor G. C. Willis, whose patients showed improvements of arteriosclerosis in leg arteries, etc. when given 500 mg vitamin C, 3 times daily. We daily get at least 3,000 mg of mixed vitamin C (with rutin and bioflavinoids) and Quercetin in supplements and fresh citrus fruits, green leafy vegetables, tomatoes and in the many fruits and vegetables we eat.

Vitamin E – Essential For Heart Health

According to Canada's Pioneer Shute brothers and scientist Dr. Richard Passwater, we all need vitamin E for the general health and proper body functioning. It's an essential vitamin for cardiovascular health. A low vitamin E level in the blood is one of the most reliable warning indicators of heart disease risk and future cardiovascular problems. *home.flash.net/~tnuckel/vitamin_e.htm*

Why is vitamin E essential? It helps prevent the red blood cells from clumping together, dissolves blood clots and increases oxygenation of blood, which improves the heart's supply of oxygen. Vitamin E dilates the capillaries, improves capillary strength and protects against cardiovascular scarring after a heart attack. It also helps provide relief from complaints of poor circulation, like leg cramps, cold feet, hands, etc. We recommend a daily allowance of 400 to 800 IU's of natural mixed vitamin E. In addition to supplements, there's a significant quantities of vitamin E in wheat germ, cold-pressed vegetable oils, organic whole grains, dark green leafy vegetables, beans, raw nuts and our favorite, raw sunflower seeds.

212

Magnesium For Your Heart, Blood & Arteries

Please be alert to the importance of magnesium. It keeps your heart, blood and arteries working together. Deficiencies in this essential mineral are often the root of many cardiovascular problems. Though magnesium naturally occurs in most raw foods, a healthy daily amount of 250 mg is hard to attain eating processed foods. Eat organic apples, apricots, avocados, bananas, nutritional yeast (brewers yeast), green leafy vegetables, garlic, beans, soybeans, soy products, raw nuts and seeds, brown rice, tofu, whole wheat and other whole grains, which are rich in magnesium. Herbs such as cayenne, alfalfa, fennel, hops, paprika and others add magnesium for your heart's health! *www.all-natural.com/bone.html*

Magnesium is vital to enzymatic activity. A deficiency can interfere with nerves and muscle impulses. When that happens, your blood pressure, heart activity and circulatory flow can be affected. Side-effects can lead to high blood pressure, cardiac arrhythmia, cardiac arrest and stress damage in arterial walls! For arrhythmia, magneseum orotate works miracles, along with calcium.

Locations in the Body Where Osteoporosis, Arthritis, Pain and Misery Hit the Hardest

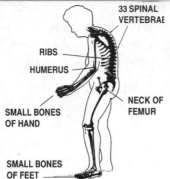

33 SPINAL VERTEBRAE

RIBS

HUMERUS

SMALL BONES OF HAND

NECK OF FEMUR

SMALL BONES OF FEET

OSTEOPOROSIS
Affects over 20 Million and Kills 300,000 Americans Annually

Boron
Miracle Trace Mineral For Healthy Bones

BORON – A trace mineral for healthier bones that also helps the body absorb more vital calcium, minerals and necessary hormones! Good sources are most vegetables, fresh and sun-dried fruits, raw nuts, soybeans and nutritional Brewer's yeast.

The U.S. Department of Agriculture's Human Nutrition Lab in Grand Forks, North Dakota, says boron is usually found in soil and in foods, but many Americans eat a diet low in boron. They conducted a 17 week study which showed a daily 3 to 6 mg. boron supplement enabled participants to reduce the loss (demineralization) of calcium, phosphorus and magnesium from their bodies. This loss is usually caused by eating processed fast foods and lots of meat, salt, sugar and fat and a dietary lack of fresh vegetables, fruits and whole grains *(www.all-natural.com)*.

213

After 8 weeks on boron, participants' calcium loss was cut 40%. It also helped double important hormone levels vital in maintaining calcium and healthy bones. Millions of women on estrogen replacement therapy for osteoporosis may want to use boron as a healthier choice. Also consider the * natural progesterone (raw yam) cream. For pain, joint support and healing use a glucosamine/chondriotin and MSM combo.

Scientific studies have shown that women benefit from a healthy lifestyle that includes some gentle sunshine and ample exercise to maintain healthier bones, combined with a low-fat, high-fiber, carbohydrate, fruit and veggie diet. This helps protect against heart disease, high blood pressure, cancer and many other ailments. I'm happy to see science now agrees with my Dad who first stated these health truths over 88 years ago!

---

* *For more hormone and osteoporosis facts read John Lee, M.D.'s book*
What Your Doctor May Not Tell You About Menopause www.johnleemd.com

Wise Heart Wisdom From Dr. James Balch*
Indications of Heart Trouble:

• Angina Pectoris: refers to the pain or feeling of tightness, pressure in the chest. This is a warning sign of impending heart attack. The pain may be mild or severe. (page 16)

• Arrhythmias: electrical disorders that disrupt the heart's natural rhythm. Palpitations happen when the heart beats out of sequence. The victim feels as if their heart is skipping beats. Studies show magnesium can correct irregular heart beats and save lives of heart patients.

• Cardiac Arrest: occurs when the heart stops beating. The blood supply is then stopped to the brain and the victim loses consciousness. Unsuspected coronary artery disease is often the cause of these attacks. Victims will experience brief dizziness followed by unconsciousness.

• Congestive Heart Failure: happens when a damaged heart becomes fatigued and is unable to pump effectively. This heart exhaustion results in fluid accumulation in the lungs, labored breathing and swelling in lower legs.

• Fibrillation: artrial fibrillation and flutter, heart palpitations or enhanced awareness of heart beating. Dizziness and fainting spells often accompany atrial fibrillation.

• Myocardial Infarction: blood clots causing a narrowed coronary artery, cutting off nutrients and oxygen to the heart for a period of time, the victim suffers a myocardial infarction or heart attack, damage to heart.

• Ischemic Heart Disease: is caused by arteriosclerosis, in which fatty deposits along the walls of the arteries obstruct blood flow to the heart. Sections of the heart muscle may die in those suffering from chronic ischemia. It can lead to angina, myocardial infarction (a coronary), cardiac arrhythmias or congestive heart failure. (page 16)

• For Ischemic Stroke: this new TPA clot buster is miraculous. Tissue Plaminogen Activator is being used by cardiologists, hospitals, emergency clinics! It breaks up clots and dissolves them in 71% of patients when administered within 3 hours of an ischemic stroke! Diagnosing stroke symptoms quickly is crucial for recovery!

Bragg Health Books were My Conversion to The Healthy Way.
– James Balch, M.D., *Author of Prescription for Nutritional Healing* *

214

A new cardiokymography (CKG) test helps detect heart disease quickly. Doctors may be able to detect "silent" heart disease when CKG is used with electrocardiograms (EKGs). A recent study revealed that EKGs alone missed 39% of heart disease cases. When CKG was added to EKGs only 8% of the cases went undetected (pages 36-37).

Some heart patients may benefit from suma herb tea. Take 3 cups of this herb tea daily with ginkgo biloba extract.

* Excerpts from *Prescription for Nutritional Healing,* By James Balch, MD Available Health Stores or if unavailable call publisher: (800) 631-8571

Healthy Heart Wisdom From Dr. Linda Page*

Bad cholesterol (LDL) carries cholesterol through the bloodstream for cell-building needs, but leaves excess behind on artery walls and in tissues (plaque). Good cholesterol (HDL) helps prevent narrowing of the artery walls by removing the excess cholesterol and moving it to the liver for excretion as bile.

Vitamin C-rich foods like tomatoes, citrus juice and apple cider vinegar greatly enhance iron absorption.

Vitamin B12 is in sea greens, seaweed, soy foods, cereals and super greens like chlorella, spirulina and barley grass. If these foods are not in your vegetarian diet, it's vital to take vitamin B12, B6 and Folic Acid.

215

Stevia: two drops = 1 tsp. of sugar in sweetness. Tests show stevia helps regulate blood sugar. In South America, stevia is sold for diabetes and hypoglycemia. Stevia helps counteract fatigue and improves digestion. (See page 170.)

Apply wet ginger-cayenne compresses to the chest to increase circulation and loosed mucous.

Heart Arrhythmia - Lifestyle and diet change are better ways to avoid arrhythmia. If your pulse is over 80 and remains that way, you should make some diet and lifestyle improvements and get further heart diagnosis.

Good Herbs For Heart Health

Ginko Biloba, Hawthorn, Cayenne, Bee Pollen, Barley Grass, Panax & Siberian Ginseng, Garlic, Ginger & Licorice Root, Wild Cherry Bark, Capsicum, Red Clover, Green Tea, Cholorlla, Scullcap, Bilberry, Evening Primrose, Pau d'Arco, Butcher's Broom, Valerian, Motherswort, Dandelion, Black Cohosh and Blessed Thistle.

Heart Disease - Herb & Supplement Therapy - In an emergency: 1 tsp cayenne powder in water or juice, or cayenne tincture (20 drops) in water may help bring a person out of a heart attack; or take liquid Carnitine as directed. Take Ascorbate or Ester C with bioflavonoids, up to 5000 mg daily to tone the heart. To improve blood flow to the heart and boost circulation to *sticky* blood take Kyolic Super Formula 106 (with garlic, vitamin E, hawthorn and cayenne pepper), red sage tea or ginko biloba extracts 2 to 3 times daily or L-Creatine, 3000 mg daily. Antioxidents strengthen and clear the cardiovascular system. Grapeseed Extract 100 mg 3 times daily or hawthorn caps. Super foods for nutritional heart therapy are royal jelly, bee pollen, siberian ginseng. Do deep breathing exercises every morning for more body oxygen and to stimulate brain activity. Remember that chlorinated/fluoridated water destroys vitamin E. Drink distilled water.

A healing protocol for heart attacks would be 800 IUs of vitamin E, 1000 mg L-Carnitine, 2000 mg each of Lysine and Arginine to cleanse the arteries. Take 240 mg daily of Ginkgo Biloba capsules to increase blood flow to the brain. Also, Hawthorn, vitamin E & Bilberry extract.

Echinacea and Goldenseal extract in combination helps flush out infectious bacteria trapped in the blocked lymph glands and blood vessels. (Keep in first aid kit.)

Periodontal disease increases the chance of a heart attack by 2.7 times. Add CoQ10 – 100 mg to your daily health program, good for teeth, gums and your heart.

A Harvard Study show men with highest anger on personality tests are three times more likely to develop heart disease. High blood pressure affect 1 in 3 of all adults in the U.S.; it is often called "the silent killer".

Olive Oil boosts healthy HDL-cholesterol levels and helps remove fats from the blood. Bragg's cold pressed organic extra virgin Olive Oil is best. (Available health stores.)

A key mineral for heart regulation is magnesium orotate. A deficiency of magnesium can contribute to hypertension, and irregular heartbeat (arrhythmia).

Healthy Healing Heart Wisdom From Dr. Linda Page:*

Sad facts: Almost 550,000 American women died from heart disease last year, over 100,000 more deaths than men. Half of all women's deaths could be attributed to heart disease. It's already climbing in this 21st Century!

Supplements are important for your heart program:

• To help cleanse arteries: Ask health stores for an oral chelation supplemtent combination. (See inside front cover.)

• Heart regulation-stability: Chlorella, magnesium, L-Carnitine, heart stabilizer hawthorn or gotu kola extracts.

• Antioxidents: Wheat germ oil raises oxygen levels 30%, Chlorella, vit. E with selenium, CoQ-10, Ginko Biloba.

• Cardio-tonics: Hawthorn extract, cayenne, garlic, Siberian ginseng extract, phycotene microclusters.

• Anti-cholesterol-blood thinning: Ginger or cayenne – ginger caps, butcher's broom, taurine, niacin and garlic.

• Healthy Blood Chemistry: Chromium Picolinate and Ester C with bioflavonoids, Folic Acid, B6 and B12.

• Preventing small strokes: CoQ-10, ascorbate or Ester C with bioflavonoids, vitamin E and Selenium and SOD.

• Calcium channel blockers: Magnesium, parsley caps and L-Carnitine and L-Taurine.

Vitamin C and E are powerful antioxidants and play a criticial role in heart health. Vitmain E is also an anticoagulant that helps keep blood platelets from clumping together so they can easily go through small capilaries. Vitamin E also protects arterial walls from free-radical damage. – Dr. Julian Whitaker

The root of the ginger plant helps lower blood pressure and cut cholesterol levels. Grate fresh ginger root over salads, vegetables, add to juices, etc. or get it powdered or in capsules at health stores. Also, drink ginger and hawthorn tea.

Foods high in antioxidants for the heart include green vegetables, citrus fruits, whole grains, carrots, squash, cantaloupe and raw unsalted nuts.

Herbs For Blood Cleansing and Normalizing

Burdock Root, Pau d'Arco, Sarsaparilla, Chaparral, Licorice Root, Alfalfa Red Clover, Green Tea, Dandelion, Sea Greens, Yellow Dock Root, Marshmallow, Hawthorn Berry, Chlorella, Barley Grass, Barberry Bark

Herbs For Circulatory Stimulation

Dandelion, Alfalfa, Sea Greens, Yellow Dock Root, Chlorella Hawthorn Berry, Marshmallow, Barley Grass, Barberry Bark
*Linda Page, N.D., Ph.D., *Healthy Healing* (www.healthyhealing.com)
Available Health Stores or call (888) 447-2939

Dr. Linda Page's Heart Rehabilitation Program*

• Add mono-unsaturates such as olive oil, avocados, nuts and seeds and essential fatty acids, flax oil, etc.

• Spinach and chard, broccoli, bananas, sea greens, molasses, cantaloupe, apricots, papayas, mushrooms, tomatoes and yams are potassium-rich foods.

• Broccoli, peas, whole grain breads, vegetables, pastas, sprouts, tofu and brown rice provide healthy complex carbohydrates. Have green garden variety salads daily!

• Enjoy kelp, sea greens, soy food products and flaxseed oil for they are rich in heart healthy omega-3 oils.

• Magnesium-rich foods regulate the heart: tofu, wheat germ, oat or rice bran, broccoli, potatoes, lima beans, spinach and chard. (See page 212 for list.)

• High fiber foods like whole grains, organic fruits and vegetables, legumes and herbs are high fiber foods that will keep your system cleaner and more balanced.

• Hawthorn, arjuna, ashwagandha and passionflowers are heart stabilizing herbs that provide immediate relief.

• Almost all heart disease can be treated and prevented with improved nutrition. Refined, high fat, high calorie foods create heart problems and natural, whole foods relieve them. Fried, salty and sugary foods, low fiber, fatty and dairy foods, red meats, processed meats, tobacco and caffeine all contribute to clogged arteries, LDL bad cholesterol, high blood pressure and heart attacks.

Take Caution Using Hormone Replacement Therapy

1) Premarin suppresses folic acid, dangerously raising homocysteine levels, a known risk factor in heart disease.

2) Tests show estrogen and contraceptive pills increase a woman's risk of heart disease, heart attack, stroke and serious blood clotting problems. (See page 213.)

3) SERMs (selective estrogen receptor modulators) protects against heart disease, but risk of blood clots increases.

* Excerpts from *Healthy Healing – By* Linda Page, N.D., Ph.D. • (888) 447-2939
See Doctor Page's informative website: *www.healthyhealing.com*

Chapter 20

Alternative Health Therapies
And Massage Techniques

Try Them – They Work Miracles!

Explore these wonderful natural methods of healing your body. Then choose the techniques best for you:

ACUPUNCTURE/ACUPRESSURE Acupuncture directs and rechannels body energy by inserting hair-thin needles (use only disposable needles) at specific points on the body. It's used for pain, backaches, migraines and general health and body dysfunctions. Used in Asia for centuries, acupuncture is safe, virtually painless and has no side effects. **Acupressure** is based on the same principles and uses finger pressure and massage rather than needles. Websites offer info – check them out. Web: acupuncture.com

CHIROPRACTIC Chiropractic was founded in Davenport, Iowa in 1885 by Daniel David Palmer. There are now schools in the U.S., and graduates are joining Health Practitioners in all nations of the world to share healing techniques. Chiropractic is popular and is the largest U.S. healing profession and benefits millions. Treatment involves soft tissue, spinal and body adjustment to free the nervous system of interferences with normal body function. Its concern is the functional integrity of the musculoskeletal system. In addition to manual methods, chiropractors use physical therapy modalities, exercise, health and nutritional guidance. Web: chiropractic.org

F. MATHIUS ALEXANDER TECHNIQUE Lessons to end the improper use of neuromuscular system and bring body posture back into balance. Eliminates psycho-physical interferences, helps release long-held tension, and aids in re-establishing muscle tone. Web: alexandertechnique.com

FELDENKRAIS METHOD Dr. Moshe Feldenkrais founded this in the late 1940s. Lessons lead to improved posture and help create ease and efficiency of movement. A great stress removal method. Web: feldenkrais.com

219

Open your mind for the doors of wisdom are never shut. – Ben Franklin

HOMEOPATHY In the 1800s, Dr. Samuel Hahnemann developed homeopathy. Patients are treated with minute amounts of substances similar to those that cause a particular disease to trigger the body's own defenses. The homeopathic principle is *like cures like.* This safe and nontoxic remedy is the #1 alternative therapy in Europe and Britain because it is inexpensive, seldom has any side effects, and often brings fast results. Web: *homeopthyhome.com*

NATUROPATHY Brought to America by Dr. Benedict Lust, M.D., this treatment uses diet, herbs, homeopathy, fasting, exercise, hydrotherapy, manipulation and sunlight. (Dr. Paul C. Bragg graduated from Dr. Lust's first School of Naturopathy in the U.S.) Practitioners work with your body to restore health naturally. They reject surgery and drugs except as a last resort. Web: *naturopathics.com*

OSTEOPATHY The first School of Osteopathy was founded in 1892 by Dr. Andrew Taylor Still, M.D. There's now 15 U.S. colleges. Treatment involves soft tissue, spinal and body adjustments that free the nervous system from interferences that can cause illness. Healing by adjustment also includes good nutrition, physical therapies, proper breathing and good posture. Dr. Still's premise: if the body structure is altered or abnormal, then proper body function is altered and can cause pain and illness. Web: *osteopathy.com*

220

REFLEXOLOGY OR ZONE THERAPY Founded by Eunice Ingham, author of "The Story The Feet Can Tell," inspired by a Bragg Health Crusade when she was 17. Reflexology helps the body by removing crystalline deposits from reflex areas (nerve endings) of feet and hands through deep pressure massage. Reflexology originated in China and Egypt and Native American Indians and Kenyans practiced it for centuries. Reflexology activates body's flow of healing and energy by dislodging deposits. Visit Eunice Ingham's web: *www.reflexology-usa.net* and *www.reflexology.org*

SKIN BRUSHING is wonderful for circulation, toning, cleansing and healing. Use a dry vegetable brush (never nylon) and brush lightly. Helps purify lymph so it's able to detoxify your blood and tissues. Removes old skin cells, uric acid crystals and toxic wastes that come up through skin's pores. Use loofah sponge for variety in shower or tub.

Alternative Health Therapies & Massage Techniques

REIKI A Japanese form of massage that means "Universal Life Energy." Reiki helps the body to detoxify, then rebalance and heal itself. Discovered in the ancient Sutra manuscripts by Dr. Mikso Usui in 1822. Web: reiki.com

ROLFING Developed by Ida Rolf in the 1930s in the U.S. Rolfing is also called structural processing and postural release or structural dynamics. It is based on the concept that distortions (accidents, injuries, falls, etc.) and the effects of gravity on the body cause upsets in the body. Rolfing helps to achieve balance and improved body posture. Methods involve the use of stretching, deep tissue massage and relaxation techniques to loosen old injuries and break bad movement and posture patterns, which can cause long-term health and body stress. Web: rolf.org

TRAGERING Founded by Dr. Milton Trager M.D., who was inspired at age 18 by Paul C. Bragg to become a doctor. It is an experimental learning method that involves gentle shaking and rocking, suggesting a greater letting go, releasing tensions and lengthening of muscles for more body health. Tragering can do miraculous healing where needed in the muscles and the entire body. Web: trager.com

221

WATER THERAPY Soothing detox shower, apply olive oil to skin, alternate hot and cold water. Massage areas while under hot, filtered spray (pages 110-112). Garden hose massage is great in summer. Hot detox tub bath (20 minutes) with cup each of Epsom salts and apple cider vinegar pulls out toxins by creating an artificial fever cleanse. Web:nmsnt.org

MASSAGE & AROMATHERAPY works two ways: the essence (smell) relaxes as does the massage. Essential oils are extracted from flowers, leaves, roots, seeds and barks. These are usually massaged into the skin, inhaled or used in a bath for their qualities to relax, soothe and heal. The oils, used for centuries to treat numerous ailments, are revitalizing and energizing for the body and mind. Example: Tiger Balm, MSM, echinacea and arnica help relieve muscle aches. Avoid skin creams and lotions with mineral oil – it clogs the skin's pores. Use these natural oils for the skin: almond, apricot kernel, avocado, soy, hemp seed and olive oils and mix with aroma essential oils: rosemary, lavender, rose, jasmine, sandalwood, lemon balm, etc. –6 oz. oil & 6 drops of an essential oil. Web: aromatherapy.net or frontierherb.com

MASSAGE – SELF Paul C. Bragg often said, "You can be your own best massage therapist, even if you have only one good hand." Near-miraculous improvements have been achieved by victims of accidents or strokes in bringing life back to afflicted parts of their own bodies by self-massage and even vibrators. Treatments can be day or night, almost continual. Self-massage also helps achieve relaxation at day's end. Families and friends can learn and exchange massages; it's a wonderful sharing experience. Remember, babies also love and thrive with daily massages – start from birth. Family pets also love the soothing, healing touch of massages. Web: amtamassage.org

MASSAGE – SHIATSU Japanese form of massage that applies pressure from the fingers, hands, elbows and even knees along the same points as acupuncture. Shiatsu has been used in Asia for centuries to relieve pain, common ills, muscle stress and to aid lymphatic circulation. Web: doubleclickd.com/Articles/shiatsu.html

MASSAGE – SPORTS An important support system for professional and amateur athletes. Sports massage: improves circulation and mobility to injured tissue, enables athletes to recover more rapidly from myofascial injury, reduces muscle soreness and chronic strain patterns. Soft tissues are freed of trigger points and adhesions, thus contributing to improvement of peak neuro-muscular functioning and athletic performance.

MASSAGE – SWEDISH One of the oldest and the most popular and widely used massage techniques. It's deep body massage soothes and promotes circulation and is a great way to loosen and relax muscles before and after exercise. Web: massage-one.com/style.html

*Author's Comment: We have personally sampled many of these alternative therapies. It's estimated that soon America's health care costs will leap over $2 trillion. It's more important than ever we be responsible for our own health! This includes seeking holistic health practitioners who are dedicated to keeping us well by inspiring us to practice prevention! These Alternative Healing Therapies are also popular and getting results: aroma, Ayurvedic, biofeedback, color, guided imagery, herbs, meditation, music, saunas, Tai Chi, yoga, etc. Explore them and be open to improving your earthly temple for a healthy, longer life. **Seek and find the best for your body, mind and soul.** – Patricia Bragg*

A Personal Message to Our Students
The Body Self-Cleans & Self-Heals When Given A Chance

It is our sincere desire that each one of our readers and students attain this precious super health and enjoy freedom from all nagging, tormenting human ailments. After studying this healthy heart program, you know that most physical problems arise from an unhealthy lifestyle that creates toxins throughout the body. Many of these trouble hot spots are years old and are mainly concentrated in the intestines, colon and organs.

We have taught you that there is no special diet for any one special ailment! The Bragg Healthy Lifestyle promotes cleansing through the eating of more organic raw fruits and vegetables combined with regular fasting. It is only through progressive cleansing that the human *cesspool* can be banished! We have told you that you will go through healing crises from time to time. During these cleansing times you might have weakness and might become discouraged! This is the time you must have great strength and faith! It is during these crises, when you feel the worst, that you are doing the greatest amount of deep detox cleansing. This is why weaklings, cry-babies and people without will-power and intestinal fortitude fail to follow this perfect Bragg Heathy Lifestyle System of Cleansing and Rejuvenation! Please be strong!

223

Weaklings want a cure that requires no effort on their part. Mother Nature and your body do not work that way! The average unfortunate sick person thinks of the Lord as a kind and forgiving Father who will allow them to enter the Garden of Eden effortlessly and unpunished for any violation of His and Mother Nature's Laws.

You can create your own Garden of Eden anywhere you live, regardless of climate! All you have to do is to purify the body of its toxic poisons by living a healthy lifestyle. You can reach a stage of health and youthfulness that you never thought was possible! You can feel ageless where your chronological age actually stands still and pathological age will make you younger! When your body is free of deadly toxic material you will reach the physical, mental, emotional and spiritual state that will give you happiness every waking hour as it adds many more youthful, active, joyous years to your life!

I am proud that my father was the first to recognize the need for a low cholesterol count over 50 years ago. He established 150 as the ideal, safe cholesterol level. Major groups, like the Mayo Clinic, have since followed his lead.

Dr. Julian Whitaker says the body needs no more salt than the natural organic sodium which occurs naturally in fresh foods. When you add table salt to your diet it can leak into cells, causing tissue swelling and cell deterioration . . . Happy this famous doctor agrees with my father and I.

Now learn what and how a temperate diet will bring great benefits along with it. In the first place, you will enjoy good health. – Horace 65 B.C.

Let Mother Nature help keep the doctor away. Researchers in the Netherlands have found that people who lovingly tend to houseplants or a small garden have significantly fewer heart attacks than people who don't. Gardening was also found to lower blood pressure.

The Heart Revolution Diet will prevent vascular disease and increase longevity. – Kilmer McCully, M.D., author, *Homocysteine Revolution* www.homocysteine.com

---

It's strange that some men will drink and eat anything put before them, but check very carefully the oil put in their car.

A higher percentage of Americans are obese than Canadians or Britons. – American Journal of Public Health

---

Many osteoporosis studies consistently conclude that vegetarians have stronger bones than meat-eaters. It shows it's healthier to avoid meat and dairy products for optimum health.

The caffeine in a single cup of coffee increases blood pressure 2 to 4 points for up to 3 hours.

It doesn't matter how much or long you've been smoking –- stop now and in one year your risk of heart disease will be cut by 70%. – Dr. Daniel Levy, *Framingham Heart Study Director*

Oat bran is just as effective at lowering cholesterol as drugs – and many, many times cheaper. – Prevention Magazine

---

Quietness and Cheerfulness is important and to give thanks at meals is most essential for health and happiness. – Oliver Wendell Homes

---

Trans fats such as margarine, solid vegetable shortening, chips and fast food french fries, are so bad for you because they are made with artificial fat that the body can't recognize and therefore has trouble burning, so it's absorbed instead to cause clogging problems. – Dr. Jack Scaff, famous cardiologist

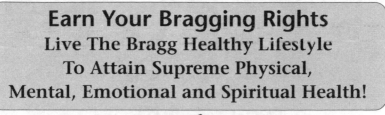

Earn Your Bragging Rights
Live The Bragg Healthy Lifestyle
To Attain Supreme Physical,
Mental, Emotional and Spiritual Health!

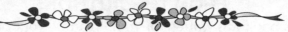

With your new awareness, understanding and sincere commitment of how to live The Bragg Healthy Lifestyle – you can now live a longer, healthier life to 120 years!

God bless you and your family and may He give you the strength, the courage and the patience to win your battle to re-enter the Healthy Garden of Eden while you are still living here on Earth with time to enjoy it all!

We have love for you and God loves you – pass it along and share this wisdom and love,

Patricia and *Paul*

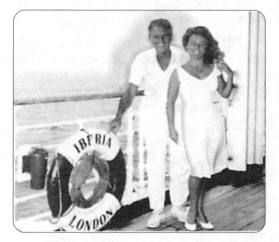

Health Crusaders Paul Bragg and daughter Patricia traveled the world spreading health, inspiring millions to renew and revitalize their health.

3 John 2 is the Bragg Crusade

The Bragg Books are written to inspire and guide you to health, fitness and longevity. Remember, the book you don't read won't help. Please re-read our books often and live The Bragg Healthy Lifestyle for a healthy, long life!

I never suspected that I would have to learn how to live – that there were specific disciplines and ways of seeing the world that I had to master before I could awaken to a simple, healthy, happy, uncomplicated life. – Dan Millman

A truly good book teaches me better than to just read it, I must soon lay it down and commence living in its wisdom. What I began by reading, I must finish by acting! – Henry David Thoreau

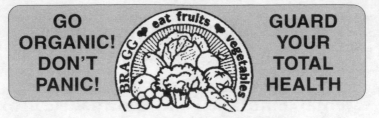

GO ORGANIC! DON'T PANIC!

BRAGG ♥ eat fruits ♥ vegetables

GUARD YOUR TOTAL HEALTH

FROM THE AUTHORS

This book was written for You! It can be your passport to a healthy, long, vital life. We in the Alternative Health Therapies join hands in one common objective – promoting a high standard of health for everyone. Healthy nutrition points the way – which is Mother Nature and God's Way. This book teaches you how to work with them, not against them. Health Doctors, therapists nurses, teachers and caregivers are becoming more dedicated than ever to keeping their patients healthy and fit. This book was written to emphasize the great needed importance of living a lifetime of healthy living, close to Mother Nature and God.

Statements in this book are scientific health findings, known facts of physiology and biological therapeutics. Paul C. Bragg practiced the natural methods of living for over 80 years with highly beneficial results, knowing that they were safe and of great value. His daughter Patricia lectured and co-authored the Bragg Books with him and continues to carry on The Bragg Health Crusades.

Paul C. Bragg and daughter Patricia express their opinions solely as Public Health Educators and Health Crusaders. They offer no cure for disease. Only the body has the ability to cure a person. Experts may disagree with some of the statements made in this book. However, such statements are considered to be factual, based on the long-time health experience of pioneers Paul C. Bragg and Patricia Bragg. If you suspect you have a medical problem, please seek alternative health professionals to help you make the healthiest, wisest and best-informed choices.

226

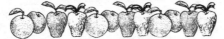

Oxygen is the main nutrient of the body. When we improve our oxygen intake, we enhance our immune system and the body's ability to detoxify and stay healthy. – Dr. Michael Schachter, Columbia University

Be sure you get calcium and magnesium together, because magnesium helps your body to metabolize calcium. Seeds, nuts and natural nut butters contain magnesium, of which you require about 300 mg. daily. Potassium is another heart – healthy mineral that lowers blood pressure and helps prevent strokes.

Your resting pulse (at times when you're not exercising) will slow down with regular exercise, a sign that it's becoming more efficient. An unfit person's resting pulse will probably be around 75. Your goal should be around 60.

Index

A

Aches & Pain, 2, 16, 38, 65, 78, 87, 152, 173, 208, 222
Acupuncture/Acupressure, 219
Adrenaline, 138
Ageing, 23, 50, 98, 160, 183, 186-188, 200-201
Alcohol, 20, 23, 32, 78, 150, 168
Allergies, 114 list, 149
Alternative Therapies, 219-222
American Heart Assocation, 24, 31, 39
Amino Acids, 117-119
Anger, 65, 72, 85, 197, 216
Angina, 16, 30, 75, 152, 154, 183, 208, 214
Angiogram (Invasive Test), 34-25, 203
Angioplasty, 35, 52
Antioxidents, inside front cover, 62, 152, 210, 217
Apple Cider Vinegar, 87, 136, 144-148, 151, 215
Arrhythmia, 37, 183, 212, 214-216
Arteries, 8, 12, 15, 46, 102, 150, 177, 199, 209, 212
Arteriosclerosis, 26, 102, 140, 199, 202
Arthritis, 209, 213-214
Aspertame, 200
Aspirin, 20
Asthma, 16-18, 47, 110-111, 144
Atherosclerosis, 15, 26, 39, 192, 199, 202-203, 208

B

Balch, Dr. James, 158, 214-215
Bee pollen, 215-216
Beta Blockers, 32
Beverages, 116, 128, 146, 151, 156
Bible Quotes, v, ix xv, 45, 47, 50, 63, 87, 161-162, 184-186
Bladder, 12
Blood, 8, 11-13, 39, 45-47, 69, 71, 75, 107, 136, 160, 217
Blood Pressure, 14, 20, 23, 29-32, 43, 54, 63, 86, 133, 183
Body, 1, 117   Bones, 52, 213
Boron, 213
Bowel movements, inside front cover, 12, 64
Bragg, Patricia, 3, 18, 21, 44, 49, 55, 62, 192, 222, 225
Bragg, Paul, i, xv, xvi, 41, 59, 67, 80, 88, 145, 160,
    220, 222, 225-226
Bragg Healthy Lifestyle, ii, 23-24, 49, 65, 97,
    101, 146, 149, 155, 160, 171, 185, 196, 208
Brain 1, 39, 63, 65, 68, 72, 107, 153, 176, 208
Breathing 67-71, 170, 220
Brewer's (nutritional) yeast 146-147, 211-213
Bright's Disease 177
By-Pass Surgery 34-35, 199

C

Caffeine (coffee), 7, 74, 76-78, 148, 168, 218, 224
Calcium, 31, 115, 130-131, 168, 202, 212-214
Cancer, 22-23, 38, 49, 72-73, 96, 126, 145, 183, 213
Capillaries, 12, 69, 209, 211
Carbohydrates, 47, 66, 82, 117, 120, 213, 218
Cardiac Arrest, 123, 212, 214
Cardiokymography (CKG), 27, 215
Cardiovascular Disease, 169, 183, 208, 212
Carrel, Dr. Alexis, 40
Cataracts, 23, 75
Cayenne (capsaicin), 209, 215
Chelation, viii, x, 199-205
Children, 30, 47-49, 69, 122, 130, 142, 165
China Project, 96
Chinese Recipes, 192-193
Chiropractic, 219
Chlorine, 210, 216
Cholesterol, 15, 20-27, 49, 59, 115-116, 120,
    124-126, 138, 140, 170, 189, 205-209, 215
Chondroitin sulfate, inside front cover, 209
Circulation, 8, 10, 13, 88-90, 95, 222
Cleansing, 156, 223
Clogging, 17, 26, 211
Clots, 15, 176, 214
Colds, 47, 158
Congestive Heart Failure, 37, 183, 214
Constipation, inside front cover, 12, 64
CoQ10, inside front cover, 183, 201, 216-217
Coronary (disease), 7, 172, 189, 214

D

Danger signals, 59
Defibrillator (AED), 123
Depression, 32, 54, 153, 208
Detoxification, 106
Diabetes, 23, 31, 49
Diastolic (blood pressure), 30, 44, 183
Dialysis, 19
Diet, American, 28
Digestion, 1, 30, 44, 136, 151, 209
Diuretics, 32
DMSO, inside front cover, 209
Doppler, 36, 49
Dribbles 12
Dropsy, 177
Drugs, 66, 220

Touch is a primal need, as necessary for growth as a food, clothing or shelter. Michelangelo knew this: when he painted God extending a hand toward Adam on the ceiling of the Sistine Chapel, he chose touch to depict the gift of life. – George H. Colt

When you sell a man a book you don't just sell him paper, ink and glue, you sell him a whole new life! There's heaven and earth in a real book, and the main purpose of books is to trap the mind into its own thinking and action. – Christopher Morley

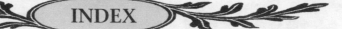

E

Echineccea, 216, 222
Echocardiography, 37
EDTA (chelation), 199-205
Electrocardiogram (EKG), 37-38, 215
Elimination, 12, 64, 106, 114, 124, 156, 161, 175, 189
Emergencies, 16, 25, 38, 69, 123, 173, 214, 216
Emphysema, 73, 75, 200
Energy, 65, 74, 219-220, 222
Enzymatic Activity, inside front cover, 212
Emotionalism, 188
Estrogen, 212-213, 218
Exercise, i, viii, 5, 37, 79-101, 141, 146, 150, 169, 214, 219-222
Eyes, 23, 75, 112, 204

F

Faith, v
Fasting, 16, 25, 49, 58, 99, 106, 155-161, 206, 220, 223
Fat (obsity), 23, 30, 40, 48-49, 54-60, 132, 141-142
Fatigue, 32
Fats (in foods), 21-28, 48, 120-124, 140, 150
Feet, 86, 90, 94-95
Fiber, 53, 154, 159, 218
Fibrillation, 123, 214   Flavoniods, 210
Flaxseed, 123-124, 146, 157, 174, 218
Fletcherizing, 151
Fluoride, 109, 216
Folic Acid (Folate), 54, 136, 153-154, 211, 218
Foods 44, 117, 129, 137, 142, 147-149
Foods to avoid list, 48, 148
Framingham Study, 16, 96
Free Radicals, 22-23, 209-210
Fruits, 31, 43, 49, 62, 82, 102, 115, 117, 124, 139, 143, 145-146, 153, 158, 193, 213

G

Garlic, 43, 56-57, 123, 136, 145, 207-208, 216
Gasteointestinal tract, 81, 136
Ginger, 215
Ginko Biloba, 207-209, 215-216
Glucosamine, inside front cover, 209, 213
Grains, 115, 120, 122, 128, 138-139, 143, 148, 150, 212
Goldenseal, 216
Gotu Kola, 208
Grapeseed Extract, 210, 216
Gums, 42, 116, 183, 210, 216

H

Habits, 77
Hardening of the arteries, 101-102, 201-202
Harvard Studies, 32, 34, 80, 216
Hawthorn Berry, 207-208, 215-217
HDL, good cholesterol, insde front cover, 22, 208, 215
Headaches, 65, 156
Healing Crisis, 156, 223
Heart Attacks, 2, 5, 9, 15-16, 20, 59, 121, 126, 141 142, 152, 172-173, 176, 194-195, 211, 215
Heart Disease, 6, 27 (list), 35, 47, 62, 85-86, 95, 121, 125, 187, 216
Heart Failure, 214
Heart Fitness Points, 169-170, 178, 182
Heart Surgery, (Transplants), 34, 170-171, 196, 206
Heartburn, 4, 151
Heimlich Maneuver, 17-18
Herbs, 136, 146, 157, 190, 207-208, 215-218
Hilton, Conrad, 55
Hippocrates, 152
Hobbies, 94
Holter Monitor, 38
Homeopathy, 220
Homeostasis, 116
Homocysteine, 39, 153-154, 211, 218, 224
Hormones, 33, 47, 138, 213-214, 218
Hospitals, 56
Hydrogenated fat, 28
Hydrotherapeutic, 95
Hyperactivity, 107
Hypertension, 29, 31, 81

I

Insomnia, 153, 163-168
Insulin, 49, 202, 204
Ischemia Strokes & Disease, 38, 214
Isoflavins, 118-119, 124, 126, 145

J

Jealosy, 72
Juices, 104, 125, 154, 158-159
Junk Foods, 48, 54, 148, 173

K

Kelp, 136, 218
Kidneys, 1, 10, 12, 19, 30, 50, 58. 83, 92, 107, 168
Killer foods, 148, 150, 190
Koop, Dr. C. Everett, 104, 149

When you can think of yesterday without regret, and of tomorrow without fear, then you are on the road to success.

Follow the steps of the godly instead, and stay on the right path, for good men enjoy life to the full. – Proverbs 2:20-21

L

Labels, 115   LaLanne, Jack and Elaine, 80
L-Carnitine, L-Creatine, 216
LDL (bad cholesterol), 22, 215
Lecithin, inside front cover, 124-126
Lemon, 136, 139, 147, 159, 167, 179, 190-191
Lentils, 54, 120, 139, 143, 147, 180
Leptin, 142
Lifestyle, 2,5-7, 20-21, 33, 35,
Lipids, 54, 128
Lipoproteins, 21-22
Liver, 21, 67, 92
Longevity, xvi, 42, 58, 185-187
Low-fat, 122
Lungs, 11, 13, 60, 68-71, 81, 93, 107
Lyon Diet Heart Study, 152

M

Magnesium, 31, 115-116, 136, 168, 212-213, 216 218, 226
Massage, 91, 167, 220-222
Mattress, 166
Meat, 21-22, 42, 54, 114, 118, 138-140, 143, 148, 190, 192, 224
Medicinal plants, 207
Meditation, prayer, 54, 67, 85, 100, 144, 194, 205
Mediterranean diet, 152
Melatonin, inside front cover, 168
Memory, 176, 208
Meridian paths, 220
Milk, 21, 26, 102, 114, 116, 122, 130-131, 140, 143, 194
Minerals, 102-103, 115-116, 124, 214, 226
Minimally Invasive Surgery, 56
MRI, 36
MSM, inside front cover, 209, 213
Mushrooms, 140, 147, 152, 154, 191, 193, 218
Myocardial infarctions, 214

N

Nature, iv   Naturopathy, 220
Nerves, 1, 3, 67, 93, 130
Niacin, inside front cover, 211, 217
Nicotine, 7, 20, 72-73, 75, 168
Nitric Oxide, 23
Nitrates, 220
Non-Invasive Test, 34-35, 203-204
Nurses Health Study, 129
Nutrition, 5, 142, 146-149, 160, 219-220, 226
Nutritional (Brewer's) yeast, 146-147, 211-213
Nuts/Nut Butters, 54, 114-115, 117, 123, 135, 139, 148, 226

O

Obesity, 23, 30, 40, 48-49, 58-61, 60, 132, 141-142, 224
Occlusion, 15
Oils, 123-124, 143, 146, 152, 157, 174, 218
Olive Oil, 124, 129, 152, 194, 216
Onions, 51, 136, 226
Organic foods, 63-64, 21, 169
Ornish, Dean, M.D. 7, 31, 33, 35
Osteoporosis, 54, 75, 98, 116, 153, 204, 213-214, 224
Overeating, 141-142
Oxygen, 11, 13, 66-71, 75, 201, 226

P

Pacemaker, 37, 177
Pain reliever, 209, 213
Pancreas, 23, 204
Page, Dr. Linda, 215-218
Penicillin, (Garlic) 34
Pep Drinks, 146
Periodontal disease, 183, 216
Pesticides, 3, 71, 113, 115, 138, 210
Phosphorus, 115
Physical education, 48-49
Physical therapy, 176
Phytochemicals, 118, 145 (chart)
Pillow, 165-166
Plaque, 205
Plasma, 47
Pollution, air & water, 70, 138
Positron Emission Tomgraphy (PET), 38
Posture, 142, 151, 219-222
Potassium, 31, 132, 181
Premarin, 213, 218
Premature ageing, 23, 186
Prevention, 4-5, 172, 177, 191
Progesterone, 213
Prostate Problems, 145
Protein, 117,   % Protein Vegetarian(list) 139
Pulse, 4, 13, 44, 114 (test), 226

R

Radiation, 210
Rage, 65, 72, 85, 197, 216
Recipes, 133, 146-147, 179-180, 184, 192-193
Refined Foods, 29, 42, 77, 116, 120, 126-127, 143, 148, 173
Reflexology (Therapy), 220
Reiki (Therapy), 222
Rejuvenation, 150, 201
Relaxation, ix, 222
Rice Casserole Recipe, 147
Russia, ii   Rutin (Vitamin), 211

Good health, generated by physical fitness is the logical starting point for the pursuit of excellence in any field. Physical vitality promotes mental vitality and thus is essential to executive achievement.
– Dr. Richard E, Dutton, University of Southern Florida

S

Salads, 147, 157, 179-180, 190-191
Salad Dressings, 137, 179, 190
Salt, 29, 132-137, 148, 224
Salt Licks, 132
Salt Tablets, 134
Saturated fats, 24, 28
Scholl, Dr., 86
Seeds, 110, 114-115, 117, 123, 135, 138, 226
Senility, 110, 208
Shakespeare, 63
Shiatsu Therapy, 222
Shoes, 86, 94-95
Shower, 91, 110-112, 222
Sitting, 92-93
Skin, 67, 93, 220
Skullcap, 168
Sleep, 13, 163-168
Smog, 70-71, 210
Smoking, 20, 23, 69, 72-77, 96, 169, 187, 224
Sodium, 115, 136-137
Soy, 116, 119, 122, 125-128, 132, 136-137,
      143, 190, 193, 213
Spasm, 16
Speech, slurred, 19
Spincter muscles, 12
Spinal Column, 69
Spock, Dr. Benjamin, 122
Stevia, 170, 215
Stress, 2-3, 28, 54, 177
Stretching, viii, 62, 89-90, 183, 222
Stroke, 19-20, 39, 102, 123, 175-177, 183, 193, 195, 217
Sunshine, 43, 213, 220
Surgery, 34, 200, 220
Sweating, 1, 93
Symptoms, 16, 29, 156, 177, 200
Systems, of the body, 219-220
Systolic (Blood pressure), 30, 44, 86

T

Taste buds 37, 137, 194
Teeth and Gums, 42, 116, 183
Tendons, 67   Tests, 35-38, 203
Therapies, 219-222
Thermographic scan, 204
Thrombosis, 15, 28, 39, 92
Tissue Plaminogen Activator (TPA), 214
Tissue rejection, 171
Tobacco, 72
Tofu, 122, 128, 143, 146, 211-212
Transplants, 170, 196
Triglycerides, inside front cover, 23, 141, 206
Tuberculosis, 137

U

Ultrasound, 36
Universal Life Energy, 222
Unsaturated fats, 28, 193
Uric acid, 138
Urination, 12, 116, 112 (exercise)

V

Varicos veins, 74
Vascular system, 50, 153, 194, 200
Vegetables, 26, 31, 43, 62, 105, 116-117, 120
      124, 129, 139, 143-145, 147, 157-158, 218
Vegetarian, 33, 54, 139 (list), 175, 191, 224
Veins, 8, 12, 46, 209
Ventricle, 10, 37
Ventricular (left) Hypertrophy, 29
Vision, 23, 75, 112, 200, 204, 210
Vitamins, 123
      A, 130, 210
      B's, 153-154, 203, 211, 214-215
      C, 74, 210-211, 215
      D, 130, 200, 210
      E, 62, 127, 129 (list), 142, 212, 216-217

W

Waistline, 60-61, 68, 141
Walking, 80-88, 170
Water, 95, 101-112, 113 (chart), 221 (therapy)
Water Fast, 158
Websites, 14, 19, 27, 35-38, 40-41, 62-63, 80, 83,
      85, 96, 98-99, 109-110, 122-123, 131, 142,
      152-153, 174, 177, 191, 198, 205-222
Weight Lifting, 80, 97-99
Wheat Germ, 125, 127, 217
Whitaker, Dr. Julian, 35, 152, 224

X

Xanthelasma, 24
Xanthoma, 24
X-Knife Sterotactic Radiosurgery, 38

Y

Youthful, 97, 195-197

Z

Zinc, 106, 123, 202
Zora Agha, 42, 50

Your Daily Habits Form Your Future

*Habits can be wrong, good or bad, healthy or unhealthy, rewarding or unrewarding.
The right or wrong habits, decisions, actions, words or deeds . . . are up to you!
Wisely choose your habits, as they can make or break your life! – Patricia Bragg*

Send for Free Health Bulletins

Patricia Bragg wants to keep in touch with you, your relatives and friends about the latest Health, Nutrition, Exercise and Longevity Discoveries. Please enclose one stamp for each USA name listed. Foreign listings send postal reply coupons.
With Blessings of Health and Thanks,

Patricia

Please print or type addresses clearly and mail to:

BRAGG HEALTH CRUSADES, Box 7, Santa Barbara, CA 93102
You can help too!
Keep the Bragg Health Crusades "Crusading" with your tax-deductible gifts.

Name _____

Address _____ Apt. No. _____

City _____ State _____ Zip _____

Phone ( ) _____ E-mail _____

Name _____

Address _____ Apt. No. _____

City _____ State _____ Zip _____

Phone ( ) _____ E-mail _____

Name _____

Address _____ Apt. No. _____

City _____ State _____ Zip _____

Phone ( ) _____ E-mail _____

Name _____

Address _____ Apt. No. _____

City _____ State _____ Zip _____

Phone ( ) _____ E-mail _____

Name _____

Address _____ Apt. No. _____

City _____ State _____ Zip _____

Phone ( ) _____ E-mail _____

Bragg Health Crusades spreading health worldwide over 88 years

BRAGG "HOW-TO, SELF-HEALTH" BOOKS

Authored by America's First Family of Health
Live Longer – Healthier – Stronger Self-Improvement Library

Qty.	Bragg Book Titles ORDER FORM Health Science ISBN 0-87790	Price	$ Total
	Apple Cider Vinegar – Miracle Health System (6 million in print)	6.95	.
	Bragg Healthy Lifestyle – Vital Living to 120 (formerly Toxicless Diet)	7.95	.
	Super Power Breathing for Super Energy and High Health	7.95	.
	Miracle of Fasting – Bragg Bible of Health for longvity & physical rejuvenation	8.95	.
	Water – The Shocking Truth (learn safest water to drink & why)	7.95	.
	Nature's Healing Eyesight Program	8.95	.
	Bragg's Gourmet Health Recipes for Super Health – 448 pages	9.95	.
	Bragg Vegetarian Recipes (new version) for Super Health	9.95	.
	Build Powerful Nerve Force (reduce fatigue, stress, anger, anxiety)	8.95	.
	Healthy Heart & Cardiovascular System – Have a fit heart at any age	8.95	.
	Healthy, Strong Feet – "Best Complete Foot Progam" – Dr. Scholl	8.95	.
	Bragg Back Fitness Program for pain-free back	7.95	.

Total Copies Prices subject to change without notice.

TOTAL BOOKS $.

USA Shipping ⟩ Please add $3 for first book, $1.00 for each additional book.

USA retail book orders over $35 add $5 only.

Canada & Foreign orders add $3 first bk, $1.50 @ add'l bk.

| CA residents add sales tax | . |
| Shipping & Handling | . |

Please Specify: ☐ Money Order ☐ Cash ☐ Check

TOTAL ENCLOSED $.
(USA Funds Only)

Charge To: ☐ Visa ☐ Master Card ☐ Discover

Credit Card Number: _ _ _ _   _ _ _ _   _ _ _ _   _ _ _ _   Card Expires: ___|___

Month   Year

MasterCard   VISA   DISCOVER   **Signature:** _____

CREDIT CARD ORDERS ONLY
CALL **(800) 446-1990**
OR FAX **(805) 968-1001**

Business office calls (805) 968-1020. We accept MasterCard Discover or VISA phone orders. Please prepare your order using this order form. It will speed your call and serve as your order record. Hours: 9 am to 4 pm Pacific Time, Monday thru Thursday.
Visit our Web Site: http://www.bragg.com & e-mail: bragg@bragg.com

Mail to: **HEALTH SCIENCE, Box 7, Santa Barbara, CA 93102 USA**

Please Print or Type – Be sure to give street & house number to facilitate delivery.   BOF-701

Name _____

Address _____   Apt. No. _____

City _____   State _____   Zip _____

Phone (   )   ● E-mail

Bragg Organic Raw Apple Cider Vinegar
With the Mother . . . Nature's Delicious, Healthy Miracle

HAVE AN APPLE HEALTHY LIFE!

– IF ? –

Your Favorite Health Store doesn't carry Bragg Products Ask them to Contact their Distributor to stock them! Or they can Call Bragg at 1-800-446-1990

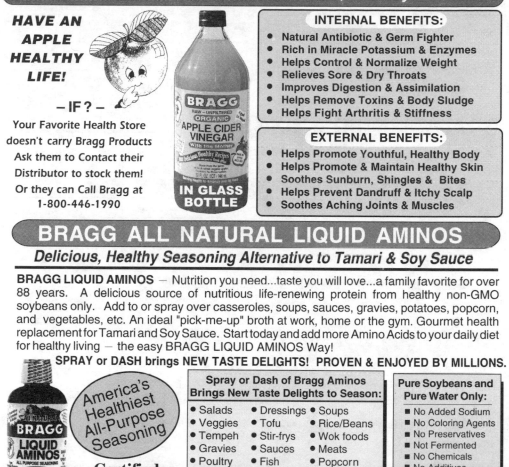

IN GLASS BOTTLE

INTERNAL BENEFITS:
- Natural Antibiotic & Germ Fighter
- Rich in Miracle Potassium & Enzymes
- Helps Control & Normalize Weight
- Relieves Sore & Dry Throats
- Improves Digestion & Assimilation
- Helps Remove Toxins & Body Sludge
- Helps Fight Arthritis & Stiffness

EXTERNAL BENEFITS:
- Helps Promote Youthful, Healthy Body
- Helps Promote & Maintain Healthy Skin
- Soothes Sunburn, Shingles & Bites
- Helps Prevent Dandruff & Itchy Scalp
- Soothes Aching Joints & Muscles

BRAGG ALL NATURAL LIQUID AMINOS
Delicious, Healthy Seasoning Alternative to Tamari & Soy Sauce

BRAGG LIQUID AMINOS – Nutrition you need...taste you will love...a family favorite for over 88 years. A delicious source of nutritious life-renewing protein from healthy non-GMO soybeans only. Add to or spray over casseroles, soups, sauces, gravies, potatoes, popcorn, and vegetables, etc. An ideal "pick-me-up" broth at work, home or the gym. Gourmet health replacement for Tamari and Soy Sauce. Start today and add more Amino Acids to your daily diet for healthy living – the easy BRAGG LIQUID AMINOS Way!

SPRAY or DASH brings NEW TASTE DELIGHTS! PROVEN & ENJOYED BY MILLIONS.

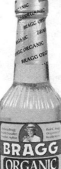

America's Healthiest All-Purpose Seasoning

Certified Non-GMO

Spray or Dash of Bragg Aminos Brings New Taste Delights to Season:			Pure Soybeans and Pure Water Only:
• Salads	• Dressings	• Soups	■ No Added Sodium
• Veggies	• Tofu	• Rice/Beans	■ No Coloring Agents
• Tempeh	• Stir-frys	• Wok foods	■ No Preservatives
• Gravies	• Sauces	• Meats	■ Not Fermented
• Poultry	• Fish	• Popcorn	■ No Chemicals
• Casseroles & Potatoes		• Macrobiotics	■ No Additives
			■ Certified Non-GMO

BRAGG ORGANIC OLIVE OIL
Extra Virgin, Unrefined, First Cold-Pressed

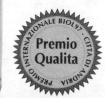

Premio Qualita

BRAGG ORGANIC OLIVE OIL – is made from a blend of 100% organically grown Arbequina and Frantoio Olives that continually provides the best quality and flavor. It's a heart healthy oil that is an antioxidant and vitamin E rich, helping to normalize cholesterol and blood pressure. Bragg Olive Oil has a delicious, smooth body with a light after taste, adding the finest flavor and aroma to salads, vegetables, pastas, pestos, sauces, sautés, potatoes and most foods – even popcorn. In 400 B.C. Hippocrates, the Father of Medicine used and wrote about the great health benefits of olive oil.

BRAGG OLIVE OIL VINAIGRETTE OR MARINADE
⅓ cup Bragg Organic Extra Virgin Olive Oil
½ cup Bragg Organic Apple Cider Vinegar
½ tsp Bragg Liquid Aminos (All-Purpose) Seasoning
1 to 2 tsp raw honey • 1 to 2 cloves garlic, minced
Pinch of Italian or French herbs

BRAGG ORGANIC APPLE CIDER VINEGAR

SIZE	PRICE	USA SHIPPING & HANDLING	AMT	$ TOTAL
16 oz.	$ 2.19 each	Please add $4 for 1st bottle and $1.50 each additional bottle		.
16 oz.	$26.28 Case/12	S/H Cost by Time Zone: CA $8. PST/MST $9. CST $13. EST $16.		.
32 oz.	$ 3.79 each	Please add $5 for 1st bottle and $2.00 each additional bottle.		.
32 oz.	$45.48 Case/12	S/H Cost by Time Zone: CA $11. PST/MST $15. CST $21. EST $27.		.
Bragg Vinegar is a food and not taxable			**Vinegar** $	.
			Shipping & Handling	.
			TOTAL $	.

BRAGG LIQUID AMINOS

SIZE	PRICE	USA SHIPPING & HANDLING	AMT	$ TOTAL
6 oz.	$ 2.98 each	Please add $3 for 1st 3 bottles – $1.25 each additional bottle.		.
6 oz.	$ 71.52 Case/24	S/H Cost by Time Zone: CA $6. PST/MST $8. CST $10. EST $12.		.
16 oz.	$ 3.95 each	Please add $4 for 1st bottle – $1.25 each additional bottle.		.
16 oz.	$47.40 Case/12	S/H Cost by Time Zone: CA $7. PST/MST $8. CST $11. EST $13.		.
32 oz.	$ 6.45 each	Please add $5 for 1st bottle – $1.50 each additional bottle.		.
32 oz.	$77.40 Case/12	S/H Cost by Time Zone: CA $9. PST/MST $12. CST $17. EST $21.		.
Bragg Aminos is a food and not taxable			**Aminos** $	.
			Shipping & Handling	.
			TOTAL $	.

BRAGG ORGANIC OLIVE OIL

SIZE	PRICE	USA SHIPPING & HANDLING	AMT	$ TOTAL
12.7 oz.	$ 6.78 each	Please add $3.20 for 1st bottle and $1.25 each additional bottle.		.
12.7 oz.	$ 81.36 Case/12	S/H Cost by Time Zone: CA $7. PST/MST $8. CST $12. EST $13.		.
Bragg Olive Oil is a food and not taxable			**Olive Oil** $	.
			Shipping & Handling	.
			TOTAL $	.

Foreign orders, please inquire on postage

Please Specify: ☐ Check ☐ Money Order ☐ Cash

Charge To: ☐ Visa ☐ MasterCard ☐ Discover

Credit Card Number: _ _ _ _ _ _ _ _ _ _ _ _ _ _ _ _   Card Expires: Month | Year

MasterCard VISA DISCOVER

Signature:

CREDIT CARD ORDERS ONLY
CALL **(800) 446-1990**
OR FAX **(805) 968-1001**

Business office calls (805) 968-1020. We accept MasterCard Discover or VISA phone orders. Please prepare your order using this order form. It will speed your call and serve as your order record. Hours: 9 am to 4 pm Pacific Time, Monday through Thursday. Visit our Web Site: http://www.bragg.com & e-mail: bragg@bragg.com

Mail to: **HEALTH SCIENCE, Box 7, Santa Barbara, CA 93102 USA**

Please Print or Type – Be sure to give street & house number to facilitate delivery.

BOF-701

Name

Address   Apt. No.

City   State

( )

Phone   Zip   E-mail